MY INSTANT POT RECIPES 2022

DELICIOUS AND EASY BUDGET-FRIENDLY RECIPES

MELANIA GREENE

Table of Contents

Hot Chicken Soup

Preparation Time: 20 minutes

Servings 5

Nutritional Values per serving: 238 Calories; 17g Fat; 5.4g Total Carbs; 16.4g Protein; 2.6g Sugars

Ingredients

- 2 tablespoons grapeseed oil
- 2 banana shallots, chopped
- 4 cloves garlic, minced
- 1 cup Cremini mushrooms, sliced
- 2 bell peppers, seeded and sliced
- 1 serrano pepper, seeded and sliced
- 2 ripe tomatoes, pureed
- 1 teaspoon porcini powder
- 2 tablespoons dry white wine
- Sea salt and ground black pepper, to your liking
- 1 teaspoon dried basil
- 1/2 teaspoon dried dill weed
- 5 cups broth, preferably homemade
- 4 chicken wings

Directions

1. Press the "Sauté" button and heat the oil. Once hot, sauté the shallots until just tender and aromatic.

2. Add the garlic, mushrooms, and peppers; cook an additional 3 minutes or until softened.
3. Now, stir in tomatoes, porcini powder, white wine, salt, and black pepper. Add the remaining ingredients and stir to combine.
4. Secure the lid. Choose "Manual" mode and High pressure; cook for 18 minutes. Once cooking is complete, use a quick pressure release.
5. Make sure to release any remaining steam and carefully remove the lid. Remove the chicken wings from the Instant Pot. Discard the bones and chop the meat.
6. Add the chicken meat back to the Instant Pot. Ladle into individual bowls and serve warm. Bon appétit!

Chicken Fillets with Bacon and Cheese

Preparation Time: 25 minutes

Servings 6

Nutritional Values per serving: 450 Calories; 24.1g Fat; 2.5g Total Carbs; 53.6g Protein; 0.2g Sugars

Ingredients

- 1 ¼ cups water
- 10 ounces Ricotta cheese, crumbled
- 6 chicken fillets
- Salt, to taste
- 1/2 teaspoon cayenne pepper
- 6 tablespoons bacon crumbles
- 4 ounces Monterey-Jack cheese
- 1 tablespoon chicken bouillon granules

Directions

1. Add water to the bottom of the Instant Pot. Add Ricotta cheese and chicken fillets; sprinkle with salt and cayenne pepper.
2. Secure the lid. Choose "Manual" mode and High pressure; cook for 18 minutes. Once cooking is complete, use a quick pressure release.
3. Now, shred the chicken with two forks and return it back to the Instant Pot. Stir in bacon crumbles,cheese, and chicken bouillon granules.

4. Place the lid back on the Instant Pot, press the "Sauté" button and cook an additional 4 minutes. Divide among serving plates and serve immediately. Bon appétit!

Mediterranean Chicken Wraps

Preparation Time: 20 minutes

Servings 6

Nutritional Values per serving: 238 Calories; 9.5g Fat; 6.1g Total Carbs; 29.1g Protein; 4.1g Sugars

Ingredients

- 1 ½ pounds chicken tenderloin, cut into 1/2-inch pieces
- Salt and black pepper, to taste
- 1 teaspoon dried oregano
- 1/2 teaspoon dried basil
- 1/2 teaspoon ground cumin
- 1 cup water
- 2 ripe tomatoes, pureed
- 2 garlic cloves, minced
- 1 tablespoon golden Greek peppers, minced
- 1 tablespoon freshly squeezed lemon juice
- 1 large-sized head lettuce
- 6 ounces Feta cheese, cubed
- 1 ounce Kalamata olives, pitted and sliced
- 2 Florina peppers, seeded and chopped

Directions

1. Add the chicken, salt, black pepper, oregano, basil, cumin, and water to your Instar Pot.
2. Secure the lid. Choose the "Manual" setting and High pressure; cook for 10 minutes. Once cooking is complete, use a natural pressure release; carefully remove the lid. Reserve the chicken.
3. Then, add tomatoes, garlic, and Greek peppers to the Instant Pot.
4. Press the "Sauté" button and cook for 6 minutes at Low pressure. Add the shredded chicken back into the Instant Pot.
5. To serve, divide the chicken mixture among lettuce leaves. Top with Feta cheese, olives, and Florina peppers. Roll up in taco-style, serve and enjoy!

Family Chicken Wings

Preparation Time: 45 minutes

Servings 6

Nutritional Values per serving: 301 Calories; 19g Fat; 3.5g Total Carbs; 27.4g Protein; 2.1g Sugars

Ingredients

- 1 ½ pounds chicken wings, bone-in, skin-on
- 1 tablespoon olive oil
- 1 tablespoon balsamic vinegar
- 1 tablespoon Shoyu sauce
- 2 tablespoons ketchup
- 1 cup water
- Sea salt, to taste
- 1/2 teaspoon cayenne pepper
- 1 cup mayonnaise
- 1 tablespoon sweet paprika

Directions

1. Place chicken wings, olive oil, balsamic vinegar, Shoyu sauce, ketchup, water, salt and cayenne pepper, and granulated garlic in a mixing dish.
2. Let it marinate for 30 minutes in the refrigerator. Secure the lid.

3. Now, press the "Manual" button. Cook the chicken wings along with their marinade for 14 minutes under High pressure.
4. Once cooking is complete, use a natural pressure release; carefully remove the lid.
5. In the meantime, mix mayonnaise with sweet paprika until it is well incorporated. Serve chicken wings with the paprika mayo for dipping. Bon appétit!

Chicken Fillets with Cheese Dip

Preparation Time: 15 minutes

Servings 4

Nutritional Values per serving: 314 Calories; 20.3g Fat; 1.7g Total Carbs; 29.9g Protein; 1.5g Sugars

Ingredients

- 1 tablespoon peanut oil
- 1 pound chicken fillets
- Salt and freshly ground black pepper, to taste
- 1/2 teaspoon dried basil
- 1 cup broth, preferably homemade
- Cheese Sauce:
- 3 teaspoons butter, at room temperature
- 1/3 cup double cream
- 1/3 cup Neufchâtel cheese, at room temperature
- 1/3 cup Gruyère cheese, preferably freshly grated
- 3 tablespoons milk
- 1/2 teaspoon granulated garlic
- 1 teaspoon shallot powder

Directions

1. Press the "Sauté" button and add peanut oil. Once hot, sear the chicken fillets for 3 minutes per side.

2. Season the chicken fillets with salt, black pepper, and basil; pour in the broth.
3. Secure the lid. Choose the "Manual" setting and cook for 6 minutes. Once cooking is complete, use a natural pressure release; carefully remove the lid.
4. Clean the Instant Pot and press the "Sauté" button. Now, melt the butter and add double cream, Neufchâtel cheese, Gruyère cheese and milk; add granulated garlic and shallot powder.
5. Cook until everything is heated through. Bon appétit!

Mexican-Style Chicken Tacos

Preparation Time: 30 minutes

Servings 6

Nutritional Values per serving: 443 Calories; 17.3g Fat; 4.6g Total Carbs; 63.7g Protein; 1.7g Sugars

Ingredients

- Low Carb Tortillas:
- 2 ounces pork rinds, crushed into a powder
- A pinch of baking soda
- A pinch of salt
- 2 ounces ricotta cheese
- 3 eggs
- 1/4 cup water
- Nonstick cooking spray

- **Chicken:**

- 1 ½ pounds chicken legs, skinless
- 4 cloves garlic, pressed or chopped
- 1/2 cup scallions, chopped
- 1 teaspoon dried basil
- 1/2 teaspoon dried thyme
- 1/2 teaspoon dried rosemary
- 1 teaspoon dried oregano
- Sea salt, to your liking

- 1/3 teaspoon ground black pepper
- 1/4 cup freshly squeezed lemon juice
- 1 cup water
- 1/4 cup dry white wine
- 1/2 cup salsa, preferably homemade

Directions

1. **To make low carb tortillas, add pork rinds, baking soda, and salt to your food processor; pulse a few times.**
2. Now, fold in the cheese and eggs; mix until well combined. Add the water and process until smooth and uniform.
3. Spritz a pancake pan with a nonstick cooking spray. Preheat the pancake pan over moderate heat.
4. Now, pour the batter into the pan and prepare like you would a tortilla. Reserve keeping the tortillas warm.
5. Then, press the "Sauté" button and cook chicken legs for 2 to 4 minutes per side; reserve. Add the garlic and scallions and cook until aromatic.
6. Add the remaining ingredients, except for salsa. Return the chicken legs back to the Instant Pot.
7. Secure the lid. Choose the "Poultry" setting and cook for 15 minutes. Once cooking is complete, use a quick pressure release; carefully remove the lid.

8. Shred the chicken with two forks and discard the bones; serve with prepared tortillas and salsa. Enjoy!

Southern Chicken Stew

Preparation Time: 25 minutes

Servings 6

Nutritional Values per serving: 453 Calories; 22.6g Fat; 5.9g Total Carbs; 53.6g Protein; 2.6g Sugars

Ingredients

- 2 slices bacon
- 6 chicken legs, skinless and boneless
- 3 cups water
- 2 chicken bouillon cubes
- 1 leek, chopped
- 1 carrot, trimmed and chopped
- 4 garlic cloves, minced
- 1/2 teaspoon dried thyme
- 1/2 teaspoon dried basil
- 1 teaspoon Hungarian paprika
- 1 bay leaf
- 1 cup double cream
- 1/2 teaspoon ground black pepper

Directions

1. Press the "Sauté" button to heat up your Instant Pot. Now, cook the bacon, crumbling it with a spatula; cook until the bacon is crisp and reserve.

2. Now, add the chicken legs and cook until browned on all sides.
3. Add the water, bouillon cubes, leeks, carrot, garlic, thyme, basil, paprika, andbay leaf; stir to combine.
4. Secure the lid. Choose the "Poultry" setting and cook for 15 minutes at High pressure. Once cooking is complete, use a natural pressure release; carefully remove the lid.
5. Fold in the cream and allow it to cook in the residual heat, stirring continuously. Ladle into individual bowls, sprinkle each serving with freshly grated black pepper and serve warm. Bon appétit!

Turkey Chowder with Swiss Chard

Preparation Time: 35 minutes

Servings 6

Nutritional Values per serving: 188 Calories; 9.2g Fat; 6.9g Total Carbs; 17.7g Protein; 3.2g Sugars

Ingredients

- 1 tablespoon canola oil
- 1 pound turkey thighs
- 1 carrot, trimmed and chopped
- 1 leek, chopped
- 1 parsnip, chopped
- 2 garlic cloves, minced
- 1 ½ quarts turkey broth
- 2 star anise pods
- Sea salt, to taste
- 1/4 teaspoon ground black pepper, or more to taste
- 1 bay leaf
- 1 bunch fresh Thai basil
- 1/4 teaspoon dried dill
- 1/2 teaspoon turmeric powder
- 2 cups Swiss chard, torn into pieces

Directions

1. Press the "Sauté" button and heat the canola oil. Now, brown turkey thighs for 2 to 3 minutes on each side; reserve.
2. Add a splash of turkey broth to scrape up any browned bits from the bottom.
3. Then, add the carrot, leek, parsnip and garlic to the Instant Pot. Sauté until they are softened.
4. Add remaining turkey broth, star anise pods, salt, black pepper, bay leaf, Thai basil, dill, and turmeric powder.
5. Secure the lid. Choose the "Soup" setting and cook for 30 minutes. Once cooking is complete, use a natural pressure release; carefully remove the lid.
6. Stir in Swiss chard while still hot to wilt leaves. Enjoy!

Instant Cheesy Chicken Drumsticks

Preparation Time: 25 minutes

Servings 5

Nutritional Values per serving: 409 Calories; 23.8g Fat; 4.8g Total Carbs; 41.7g Protein; 2.4g Sugars

Ingredients

- 1 tablespoon olive oil
- 5 chicken drumsticks
- 1/2 teaspoon marjoram
- 1/2 teaspoon thyme
- 1 teaspoon shallot powder
- 2 garlic cloves, minced
- 1/2 cup chicken stock
- 1/4 cup dry white wine
- 1/4 cup full-fat milk
- 6 ounces ricotta cheese
- 4 ounces cheddar cheese
- 1/4 teaspoon ground black pepper
- 1/2 teaspoon cayenne pepper
- Sea salt, to taste

Directions

1. Press the "Sauté" button and heat the oil. Once hot, brown chicken drumsticks for 3 minutes; turn the chicken over and cook an additional 3 minutes,
2. Now, add marjoram, thyme, shallot powder, garlic, chicken stock, wine, and milk.
3. Secure the lid. Choose the "Manual" setting and cook for 15 minutes. Once cooking is complete, use a natural pressure release; carefully remove the lid.
4. Shred the chicken meat and return to the Instant Pot. Press the "Sauté" button and stir in ricotta cheese, cheddar cheese, black pepper, and cayenne pepper.
5. Cook for a couple of minutes longer or until the cheese melts and everything is heated through.
6. Season with sea salt, taste and adjust the seasonings. Bon appétit!

Spicy Chicken Wingettes

Preparation Time: 1 hour 15 minutes

Servings 6

Nutritional Values per serving: 296 Calories; 22.5g Fat; 6.9g Total Carbs; 10.8g Protein; 3.3g Sugars

Ingredients

- 10 fresh cayenne peppers, trimmed and chopped
- 3 garlic cloves, minced
- 1 ½ cups white vinegar
- 1/2 teaspoon black pepper
- 1 teaspoon sea salt
- 1 teaspoon onion powder
- 12 chicken wingettes
- 2 tablespoons olive oil
- Dipping Sauce:
- 1/2 cup mayonnaise
- 1/2 cup sour cream
- 1/2 cup cilantro, chopped
- 2 cloves garlic, minced
- 1 teaspoon smoked paprika

Directions

1. Place cayenne peppers, 3 garlic cloves, white vinegar, black pepper, salt, and onion powder in a container.

Add chicken wingettes, and let them marinate, covered, for 1 hour in the refrigerator.

2. Add the chicken wingettes, along with the marinade and olive oil to the Instant Pot.
3. Secure the lid. Choose the "Manual" setting and cook for 6 minutes. Once cooking is complete, use a quick pressure release; carefully remove the lid.
4. In a mixing bowl, thoroughly combine mayonnaise, sour cream, cilantro, garlic, and smoked paprika.
5. Serve warm chicken with the dipping sauce on the side. Bon appétit!

Turkey Legs Delight

Preparation Time: 40 minutes

Servings 6

Nutritional Values per serving: 339 Calories; 19.3g Fat; 1.3g Total Carbs; 37.7g Protein; 0.4g Sugars

Ingredients

- 3 tablespoons sesame oil
- 2 pounds turkey legs
- Sea salt and ground black pepper, to your liking
- A bunch of scallions, roughly chopped
- 1 ½ cups turkey broth

Directions

1. Press the "Sauté" button and heat the sesame oil. Now, brown turkey legs on all sides; season with salt and black pepper.
2. Add the scallions and broth.
3. Secure the lid. Choose the "Manual" setting and cook for 35 minutes. Once cooking is complete, use a natural pressure release; carefully remove the lid.
4. You can thicken the cooking liquid on the "Sauté" setting if desired. Serve warm.

Old-Fashioned Paprikash

Preparation Time: 25 minutes

Servings 6

Nutritional Values per serving: 402 Calories; 31.7g Fat; 6.1g Total Carbs; 21g Protein; 3.1g Sugars

Ingredients

- 1 tablespoon lard, at room temperature
- 1 ½ pounds chicken thighs
- 1/2 cup tomato puree
- 1 ½ cups water
- 1 yellow onion, chopped
- 1 large-sized carrot, sliced
- 1 celery stalk, diced
- 2 garlic cloves, minced
- 2 bell peppers, seeded and chopped
- 1 Hungarian wax pepper, seeded and minced
- 1 teaspoon cayenne pepper
- 1 tablespoon Hungarian paprika
- 1 teaspoon coarse salt
- 1/2 teaspoon ground black pepper
- 1/2 teaspoon poultry seasoning
- 6 ounces sour cream
- 1 tablespoon arrowroot powder

- 1 cup water

Directions

1. Press the "Sauté" button to heat up the Instant Pot. Now, melt the lard until hot; sear the chicken thighs for 2 to 3 minutes per side.
2. Add the tomato puree, 1 ½ cups of water, onion, carrot, celery, garlic, peppers, and seasonings.
3. Secure the lid. Choose the "Manual" setting and cook for 20 minutes at High pressure. Once cooking is complete, use a quick pressure release; carefully remove the lid.
4. In the meantime, thoroughly combine sour cream, arrowroot powder and 1 cup of water; whisk to combine well.
5. Add the sour cream mixture to the Instant Pot to thicken the cooking liquid. Cook for a couple of minutes on the residual heat.
6. Ladle into individual bowls and serve immediately.

Medley with Chicken and Mushrooms

Preparation Time: 20 minutes

Servings 8

Nutritional Values per serving: 222 Calories; 12g Fat; 2.5g Total Carbs; 24.6g Protein; 1g Sugars

Ingredients

- 2 teaspoons olive oil
- 2 pounds chicken breast halves, cubed
- 1 teaspoon cayenne pepper
- 1 teaspoon onion powder
- 1/2 teaspoon porcini powder
- Sea salt, to taste
- 1/4 teaspoon freshly ground black pepper, or more to taste
- 1 cup white mushrooms, thinly sliced
- 1 parsnip, chopped
- 4 garlic cloves, minced
- 2 cups vegetable broth
- 2 bay leaves
- 1/2 cup half-and-half cream
- 2 heaping tablespoons fresh cilantro

Directions

1. Press the "Sauté" button to heat up the Instant Pot. Now, heat the oil until sizzling. Then, cook the chicken breast for 4 to 6 minutes, turning them over a few times.
2. Add cayenne pepper, onion powder, porcini powder, salt, black pepper, and white mushrooms. Continue to sauté until they are fragrant.
3. Now, stir in parsnip, garlic, broth, and bay leaves.
4. Secure the lid. Choose the "Manual" setting and cook for 10 minutes at High pressure. Once cooking is complete, use a quick pressure release; carefully remove the lid.
5. Add half-and-half cream and stir until the cooking liquid is slightly thickened. Serve garnished with fresh cilantro. Bon appétit!

Instant Chicken Teriyaki

Preparation Time: 15 minutes

Servings 6

Nutritional Values per serving: 326 Calories; 13.2g Fat; 3.1g Total Carbs; 45.6g Protein; 0.7g Sugars

Ingredients

- 1/3 cup coconut aminos
- 1/4 cup rice wine vinegar
- 3 tablespoons Mirin
- 8 drops liquid stevia
- 1 tablespoon cornstarch
- 1/3 cup water
- 2 tablespoons olive oil
- 2 pounds chicken legs, boneless and skinless
- 1 teaspoon garlic powder
- 1 teaspoon ginger powder
- Sea salt and black pepper, to taste
- 1/2 teaspoon sweet paprika
- 2/3 cup chicken stock

Directions

1. Press the "Sauté" button to heat up your Instant Pot. Now, add the coconut aminos, vinegar, Mirin,liquid stevia, and cornstarch; whisk to combine well.

2. Now, pour in water and cook, bringing to a boil; cook until the liquid is thickened; reserve teriyaki sauce.
3. Wipe down the Instant Pot with a damp cloth; then, heat olive oil and cook the chicken until browned. Add garlic powder andginger powder.
4. Season with salt, black pepper, and paprika.
5. Add chicken stockand 2/3 of teriyaki sauce; stir to combine. Secure the lid. Choose the "Manual" setting and cook for 10 minutes.
6. Once cooking is complete, use a natural pressure release; carefully remove the lid. Serve with the remaining 1/3 of teriyaki sauce and enjoy!

Lazy Chicken Carnitas

Preparation Time: 20 minutes

Servings 8

Nutritional Values per serving: 294 Calories; 15.4g Fat; 2.8g Total Carbs; 35.2g Protein; 1.3g Sugars

Ingredients

- 3 pounds whole chicken, cut into pieces
- 3 cloves garlic, pressed
- 1 guajillo chili, minced
- 1 tablespoon avocado oil
- 1/3 cup roasted vegetable broth
- Sea salt, to taste
- 1/2 teaspoon ground bay leaf
- 1/3 teaspoon cayenne pepper
- 1/2 teaspoon paprika
- 1/3 teaspoon black pepper
- 1 cup crème fraiche, to serve
- 2 heaping tablespoons fresh coriander, chopped

Directions

1. Place all of the above ingredients, except for crème fraiche and fresh coriander, in the Instant Pot.

2. Secure the lid. Choose the “Poultry” setting and cook for 15 minutes. Once cooking is complete, use a quick pressure release; carefully remove the lid.
3. Shred the chicken with two forks and discard the bones.Add a dollop of crème fraiche to each serving and garnish with fresh coriander. Enjoy!

Tasty Chicken Goulash

Preparation Time: 25 minutes

Servings 6

Nutritional Values per serving: 353 Calories; 19.5g Fat; 6.5g Total Carbs; 34.3g Protein; 4.3g Sugars

Ingredients

- 1 tablespoon olive oil
- 2 pounds chicken breast halves, boneless and skinless
- 2 small-sized shallots, chopped
- 1 teaspoon garlic paste
- 1 cup milk
- 2 ripe tomatoes, chopped
- 1 teaspoon curry powder
- 1 tablespoon tamari sauce
- 1 tablespoon balsamic vinegar
- 2 tablespoons vermouth
- Sea salt, to taste
- 1/2 teaspoon cayenne pepper
- 1/3 teaspoon black pepper
- 1/2 teaspoon hot paprika
- 1/2 teaspoon ginger, freshly grated
- 1 celery stalk with leaves, chopped
- 1 bell pepper, chopped

- 1 tablespoon flaxseed meal

Directions

1. Press the "Sauté" button to heat up the Instant Pot. Now, add olive oil. Once hot, sear the chicken breast halves for 3 to 4 minutes per side.
2. Add the shallots, garlic, milk, tomatoes, curry powder, tamari sauce, vinegar, vermouth, salt, cayenne pepper, black pepper, hot paprika, ginger, celery and bell pepper to the Instant Pot; stir to combine well.
3. Secure the lid. Choose the "Meat/Stew" setting and cook for 20 minutes at High pressure. Once cooking is complete, use a quick pressure release; carefully remove the lid.
4. Add flaxseed meal and continue stirring in the residual heat. Ladle into serving bowls and enjoy!

Turkey Meatloaf with Parmigiano-Reggiano

Preparation Time: 35 minutes

Servings 6

Nutritional Values per serving: 449 Calories; 29.7g Fat; 6.1g Total Carbs; 36.2g Protein; 3.2g Sugars

Ingredients

- 2 pounds ground turkey
- 2/3 cup pork rind crumbs
- 1/2 cup Parmigiano-Reggiano, grated
- 1 tablespoon coconut aminos
- 2 eggs, chopped
- Sea salt, to taste
- 1/4 teaspoon ground black pepper
- 1 yellow onion, peeled and chopped
- 2 garlic cloves, minced
- 4 ounces tomato paste
- 1 tablespoon Italian seasoning
- 1/2 cup tomato sauce
- 1 cup water
- 1 teaspoon mustard powder
- 1/2 teaspoon chili powder

Directions

1. Prepare your Instant Pot by adding a metal rack and 1 ½ cups of water to the bottom of the inner pot.
2. In a large mixing bowl, thoroughly combine ground turkey with pork rind crumbs, Parmigiano-Reggiano,coconut aminos, eggs, salt, black pepper, onion, garlic, tomato paste, Italian seasoning.
3. Shape this mixture into a meatloaf; lower your meatloaf onto the metal rack.
4. Then, in a mixing bowl, thoroughly combine tomato sauce with water, mustard and chili powder. Spread this mixture over the top of your meatloaf.
5. Secure the lid. Choose the "Meat/Stew" setting and cook for 20 minutes at High pressure. Once cooking is complete, use a natural pressure release; carefully remove the lid.
6. Afterwards, place your meatloaf under the preheated broiler for 5 minutes. Allow the meatloaf to rest for 6 to 8 minutes before slicing and serving.Bon appétit!

Southern Turkey Soup

Preparation Time: 20 minutes

Servings 4

Nutritional Values per serving: 429 Calories; 26.2g Fat; 6.7g Total Carbs; 40.2g Protein; 3.1g Sugars

Ingredients

- 2 teaspoons coconut oil
- 2 onions, chopped
- 2 garlic cloves, finely chopped
- 1/2 teaspoon freshly grated ginger
- 2 tomatoes, chopped
- 1 celery stalk with leaves, chopped
- 1 teaspoon dried basil
- 1/2 teaspoon dried rosemary
- 1 bay leaf
- 1/4 teaspoon freshly ground black pepper
- 1/2 teaspoon red pepper flakes, crushed
- Sea salt, to taste
- 3 turkey thighs
- 4 cups roasted vegetable broth
- 1/4 cup fresh parsley,finely minced

Directions

1. Press the "Sauté" button to heat up the Instant Pot. Now, heat the oil. Cook the onion and garlic until softened and aromatic.
2. Add grated ginger, tomatoes, celery, basil, rosemary, bay leaf, black pepper, red pepper, salt, turkey thighs and vegetable broth.
3. Secure the lid. Choose the "Manual" setting and cook for 15 minutes at High pressure. Once cooking is complete, use a quick pressure release; carefully remove the lid.
4. Remove turkey thighs from the soup; discard the bones, shred the meat and return it to the Instant Pot.
5. Add fresh parsley and stir well. Serve in individual bowls. Bon appétit!

Thai-Style Chicken

Preparation Time: 15 minutes

Servings 4

Nutritional Values per serving: 192 Calories; 7.5g Fat; 5.4g Total Carbs; 25.2g Protein; 2.2g Sugars

Ingredients

- 1 tablespoon coconut oil
- 1 pound chicken, cubed
- 1 shallot, peeled and chopped
- 2 cloves garlic, minced
- 1 teaspoon fresh ginger root, julienned
- 1/3 teaspoon cumin powder
- 1 teaspoon Thai chili, minced
- 1 cup vegetable broth, preferably homemade
- 1 tomato, peeled and chopped
- 1/3 cup coconut milk, unsweetened
- 1 teaspoon Thai curry paste
- 2 tablespoons tamari sauce
- 1/2 cup sprouts
- Salt and freshly ground black pepper, to taste

Directions

1. Press the "Sauté" button to heat up the Instant Pot. Now, heat the coconut oil. Cook the chicken for 2 to 3 minutes, stirring frequently; reserve.
2. Then, in pan drippings, cook the shallot and garlic until softened; add a splash of vegetable broth, if needed.
3. Add ginger, cumin powder and Thai chili and cook until aromatic or 1 minute more.
4. Now, stir in vegetable broth, tomato, coconut milk, Thai curry paste, and tamari sauce.
5. Secure the lid. Choose the "Manual" setting and cook for 10 minutes under High pressure. Once cooking is complete, use a quick pressure release; carefully remove the lid.
6. Afterwards, add sprouts, salt, and black pepper and serve immediately. Bon appétit!

Chicken Thighs with Green Beans and Potatoes

Prep Time: 8 Mins

Total Time: 25 Mins

Serving: 6

Ingredients:

- 2 pounds Chicken Thighs
- 1 pound Green Beans
- 1 pound Potatoes, peeled and halved
- Juice of 1 Lemon
- 2 tbsp Olive Oil
- 1 tbsp Ghee
- ½ cup Chicken Stock
- 1 tsp mixed Herbs
- 1 tsp minced Garlic

Direction

1. Set your Instant Pot to SAUTE and melt the ghee along with the olive oil in it.
2. Add garlic and cook for 1 minute.
3. Add the chicken thighs and cook them on all sides, until they become golden.
4. Stir in the lemon juice and herbs and cook for an additional minute.

5. Add the remaining ingredients and stir well to combine.
6. Close the lid and set the IP to MANUAL.
7. Cook for 15 minutes on HIGH.
8. Release the pressure quickly.
9. Serve and enjoy!

Nutritional Values per serving:

Calories 500

Total Fats 27g

Carbs: 19g

Protein 45g

Dietary Fiber: 3g

Quick and Easy Garlic Shredded Chicken

Prep Time: 5 Mins

Total Time: 25 Mins

Serving: 4

Ingredients:

- 1 tsp Garlic Powder
- 1 ¾ pounds Chicken Breasts
- ¼ tsp Black Pepper
- 1 cup Homemade Chicken Broth

Direction

1. Simply dump all of the ingredients in the Instant Pot.
2. Give the mixture a good stir and put the lid on.
3. Turn it clockwise to seal.
4. Set the IP to MANUAL.
5. Cook on HIGH for 20 minutes.
6. Do a quick pressure release and open the lid.
7. Shred the chicken inside the pot with 2 forks.
8. Serve and enjoy!

Nutritional Values per serving:

Calories 430

Total Fats 17g

Carbs: 0g

Protein 45g

Dietary Fiber: 0g

The Ultimate Mexican Chicken

Prep Time: 5 Mins

Total Time: 25 Mins

Serving: 6

Ingredients:

- 2 pounds Chicken Breasts
- Juice of 1 Lime
- 1 Jalapeno, seeded and diced
- ½ tsp Chili Powder
- ½ tsp Cumin
- 1 Green Bell Pepper, diced
- 1 Red Bell Pepper, diced
- 10 ounces Tomatoes, diced
- 1 Red Onion, diced
- 1 tbsp Olive Oil
- Pinch of Black Pepper

Direction

1. Set the IP to SAUTE and add the olive oil.
2. When sizzling, add the onion and peppers and cook for 3-4 minutes, until soft.
3. Add the rest of the ingredients.
4. Stir to combine and close the lid.
5. Set the Instant Pot to MANUAL.

6. Cook the chicken for 15 minutes on HIGH pressure.
7. Do a quick pressure release and open the lid.
8. Shred the chicken with two forks and stir to combine. This step is optional, you can serve the chicken as it is and garnish with the cooking liquid and veggies on top.
9. Enjoy!

Nutritional Values per serving:

Calories 340

Total Fats 14g

Carbs: 10g

Protein 45g

Dietary Fiber: 2g

Instant Rotisserie Chicken

Prep Time: 5 Mins

Total Time: 40 Mins

Serving: 4

Ingredients:

- 1 Whole Chicken About 2 ½ - 3 lb
- 1 ½ tbsp Olive Oil
- 1 cup Homemade Chicken Broth
- 1 tsp Smoked Paprika
- 1 tsp Garlic Powder

Direction

1. Wash the chicken well and pat dry with some paper towels.
2. In a small bowl, combine the paprika, garlic powder, and oil.
3. Rub this mixture into the chicken.
4. Set your Instant Pot to SAUTE and place the chicken inside.
5. Sear on all sides, until it turns golden.
6. Pour the broth around the chicken and close the lid.
7. Set the IP to MANUAL and cook on HIGH for 25 minutes.
8. Release the pressure quickly.

9. Let sit for 10 minutes before serving.
10. Enjoy!

Nutritional Values per serving:

Calories 585

Total Fats 20g

Carbs: 0.7g

Protein 95g

Dietary Fiber: 0.3g

Turkey with Leeks and Mushrooms

Prep Time: 8 Mins

Total Time: 25 Mins

Serving: 6

Ingredients:

- 2 pounds Turkey Breasts, cut into large pieces
- 2 tbsp Arrowroot
- ½ cup Homemade Chicken Broth
- ½ cup Almond Milk
- 2 Leeks, sliced
- 4 tbsp Ghee
- 1 ¼ pounds Mushrooms, sliced
- ¼ tsp Garlic Powder
- ¼ tsp Black Pepper

Direction

1. Season the turkey with garlic powder and pepper.
2. Set your IP to SAUTE and add the ghee.
3. When melted, add the turkey pieces and cook until they are no longer pink. Transfer them to a plate.
4. Add the leeks and mushrooms to the IP and cook for 3 minutes.
5. Return the turkey to the pot and pour the broth over.
6. Close the lid and cook for 8 minutes on HIGH.

7. Release the pressure naturally.
8. Whisk together the almond milk and arrowroot and stir into the pot.
9. Cook on SAUTE until thickened.
10. Serve and enjoy!

Nutritional Values per serving:

Calories 555

Total Fats 24g

Carbs: 37g

Protein 50g

Dietary Fiber: 3g

Chicken with Onion and Green Olives

Prep Time: 5 Mins

Total Time: 20 Mins

Serving: 4

Ingredients:

- 4 Chicken Breasts
- 1 can Green Olives, pitted
- ½ cup Red Onion, sliced
- 1 cup Homemade Chicken Broth
- 2 tbsp Ghee
- 2 tbsp Lemon Juice
- Pinch of Pepper

Direction

1. Set your Instant Pot to SAUTE and add the ghee.
2. When melted, add the chicken and brown on all sides.
3. Add the rest of the ingredients and put the lid on.
4. Set the Instant Pot to MANUAL and cook on HIGH for 10 minutes.
5. Do a quick pressure release.
6. Serve and enjoy!

Nutritional Values per serving:

Calories 500

Total Fats 34g

Carbs: 2g

Protein 44g

Dietary Fiber: 0.5g

Juicy and Fall-off-Bone Drumsticks

Prep Time: 5 Mins

Total Time: 45 Mins

Serving: 3

Ingredients:

- 6 Chicken Drumsticks
- ½ Bell Pepper, diced
- 2 tsp minced Garlic
- 1 tbsp Olive Oil
- 2 cups Water
- ½ Red Onion, diced
- 2 tbsp Tomato Paste
- Pinch of Pepper

Direction

1. Set your IP to SAUTE and heat the olive oil in it.
2. Add the onions and pepper and cook for 3 minutes.
3. Add the garlic and cook for an additional minute.
4. Place the drumsticks inside.
5. Whisk together the tomato paste and water and pour the mixture over the drumsticks.
6. Put the lid on and seal.
7. Set the IP to MANUAL.
8. Cook on HIGH for 15 minutes.

9. Let the pressure drop on its own.
10. Serve and enjoy!

Nutritional Values per serving:

Calories 450

Total Fats 27g

Carbs: 5.3g

Protein 42g

Dietary Fiber: 1.4g

Slow-Cooked Turkey

Prep Time: 15 Mins

Total Time: 4 hours and 15 Mins

Serving: 4

Ingredients:

- 1 ½ pounds Turkey Breasts
- 1 tbsp Organic Dijon Mustard
- 2 tbsp Olive Oil
- 2 tsp Smoked Paprika
- 1 tsp minced Garlic
- Pinch of Black Pepper
- 1 cup Homemade Chicken Broth

Direction

1. Set your Instant Pot to SAUTE and add the oil to it.
2. When hot and sizzling, add the turkey and cook until it becomes brown.
3. Whisk together ½ of the broth and the rest of the ingredients and pour over the turkey.
4. Close the lid and set the IP to SLOW COOK.
5. Cook for 2 hours.
6. Do a quick pressure release and pour the remaining broth over.
7. Seal the lid again and cook for another 2 hours.

8. Do a quick pressure release.
9. Serve and enjoy!

Nutritional Values per serving:

Calories 400

Total Fats 30g

Carbs: 2.5g

Protein 40g

Dietary Fiber: 0.5g

Mediterranean Chicken Wings

Prep Time: 15 Mins

Total Time: 10 Mins

Serving: 4

Ingredients:

- 12 Chicken Wings
- 2 tsp Tarragon
- 1 tbsp Oregano
- 6 tbsp Homemade Chicken Broth
- ¼ cup Homemade Chicken Broth
- 2 tbsp Olive Oil
- 1 tbsp Garlic Puree
- 1 tbsp Basil
- Pinch Pepper
- 1 cup of Water

Direction

1. Pour the water into the Instant Pot and lower the rack.
2. In a bowl, combine the remaining ingredients.
3. Let sit for 15 minutes.
4. Transfer the chicken wings to a baking dish.
5. Place the dish on the rack and close the lid of the IP.
6. Set the Instant Pot to MANUAL and cook for 10 minutes on HIGH.

7. Do a quick pressure release.
8. Serve and enjoy!

Nutritional Values per serving:

Calories 160

Total Fats 13g

Carbs: 0.6g

Protein 11g

Dietary Fiber: 0g

Green Chicken

Prep Time: 8 Mins

Total Time: 20 Mins

Serving: 4

Ingredients:

- 1 1/3 pounds Chicken Breasts, cubed
- 1 cup chopped Spinach
- 1/3 cup Basil Leaves
- 1/3 cup Coconut Cream
- 2/3 cup Homemade Chicken Broth
- 1 tsp minced Garlic
- 1 tbsp Olive Oil

Direction

1. Heat the oil in the Instant Pot on SAUTE.
2. Add the garlic and cook for 1 minute.
3. Add the chicken and cook until it is no longer pink.
4. Stir in the rest of the ingredients.
5. Put the lid on and seal.
6. Set the IP to MANUAL.
7. Cook on HIGH for 8 minutes.
8. Do a quick pressure release.
9. Serve and enjoy!

Nutritional Values per serving:

Calories 320

Total Fats 14g

Carbs: 4g

Protein 35g

Dietary Fiber: 1g

Juicy Herbed Turkey Breasts

Prep Time: 10 Mins

Total Time: 20 Mins

Serving: 3

Ingredients:

- 1 pound Turkey Breasts
- ¼ tsp Oregano
- ¼ tsp Thyme
- 2 tbsp chopped Basil
- 1 tbsp chopped Parsley
- Pinch of Pepper
- ¼ tsp Garlic Powder
- 1 tbsp Olive Oil
- 1 cup Water

Direction

1. Heat the oil in the IP on SAUTE.
2. Add the turkey and cook until it becomes browned on all sides.
3. Stir in the herbs and spices and pour the water over.
4. Close the lid and set the Instant Pot to MANUAL.
5. Cook on HIGH for 10 minutes.
6. Do a quick pressure release.
7. Serve as desired and enjoy!

Nutritional Values per serving:

Calories 320

Total Fats 15g

Carbs: 0g

Protein 40g

Dietary Fiber: 0g

Chicken Spaghetti Squash with Shitakes

Prep Time:8 Mins

Total Time: 40 Mins

Serving: 6

Ingredients:

- 1 cup sliced Shitake Mushrooms
- 2 pounds Chicken Breasts, chopped
- 1 Spaghetti Squash
- 1 cup Homemade Chicken Broth
- 1 tbsp Arrowroot
- 1 cup Water
- 1 tbsp Coconut Oil

Direction

1. Pour the water into the IP.
2. Place the spaghetti squash inside the steamer basket and lower it into the IP.
3. Close the lid and set the IP to MANUAL.
4. Cook for 20 minutes on HIGH.
5. Do a quick pressure release and set aside to cool.
6. Discard the cooking liquid and wipe the IP clean.
7. Set the IP to SAUTE and melt the coconut oil inside.
8. Add the chicken and cook until it becomes golden.
9. Add the rest of the ingredients and close the lid.

10. Cook on HIGH for 8 minutes.
11. Meanwhile, scrape out the flesh of the squash with a fork, into spaghetti-like strings.
12. Do a quick pressure release and open the lid.
13. Stir in the spaghetti.
14. Serve and enjoy!

Nutritional Values per serving:

Calories 260

Total Fats 12g

Carbs: 4g

Protein 22g

Dietary Fiber: 0g

Thai Peanut Chicken

Prep Time: 5 Mins

TotalTime: 33 Mins

Serving: 6

Ingredients:

- 1 ½ cups toasted peanuts
- 1 ½ lb. chicken breasts
- 2 cloves of garlic, minced
- Salt and pepper to taste
- 2 tbsp. chopped scallions for garnish

Directions

1. Place 1 cup of toasted peanuts in a food processor and pulse until smooth. This will serve as your peanut butter. For the remaining half cup of peanut, chop until fine. Set aside.
2. Press the Sauté button on the Instant Pot and place the chicken breasts and garlic. Keep on stirring for 3 minutes until the meat has turned lightly golden.
3. Season with salt and pepper to taste.
4. Pour the peanut butter that you have prepared earlier. Give a good stir and pour a cup of water.
5. Close the lid and seal off the vent.

6. Press the Manual button and adjust the cooking time to 25 minutes.
7. Do natural pressure release.
8. Garnish with chopped nuts and scallions before serving.

Calories:575; Total Fat: 34.8g; Carbs: 2.5g; Dietary Fiber: 0.2g; Protein:42g

Thai Goose with Basil

Prep Time: 10 Mins

Total Time: 40 Mins

Serving: 4

Ingredients:

- 2 tbsp minced Chilies
- 2 tbsp Coconut Oil
- 2 tsp minced Garlic
- 1 tsp minced Ginger
- 2 cups Goose Cubes
- ¼ cup chopped Basil
- 2 tbsp Coconut Aminos
- 1 ½ cups Water

Direction

1. Set your Instant Pot to SAUTE and add half of the coconut oil to it.
2. When melted, add the goose and cook until it becomes browned.
3. Transfer the goose to a baking dish.
4. Add the rest of the ingredients, except the water, to the dish and stir to combine.
5. Pour the water into the IP and lower the trivet.
6. Place the baking dish on the trivet and close the lid.

7. Cook on MANUAL for 10 minutes.
8. Do a quick pressure release.
9. Serve and enjoy!

Nutritional Values per serving:

Calories 190

Total Fats 9g

Carbs: 2g

Protein 27g

Dietary Fiber: 1g

Coconut Kale Chicken

Prep Time: 3 Mins

Total Time: 30 Mins

Serving: 4

Ingredients:

- 1 ½ pounds Chicken Breasts, chopped
- ½ cup canned diced Tomatoes
- ¾ cup Coconut Milk
- 1 cup chopped Kale
- 1 Garlic Clove, minced
- ¼ tsp Onion Powder
- ¼ tsp Paprika
- Pinch of Pepper
- 2/3 cup Homemade Chicken Stock
- ½ tsp Oregano
- 1 tbsp Olive Oil

Direction

1. Heat the oil in the Instant Pot on SAUTE.
2. Add the garlic and cook for 30 seconds.
3. Add chicken, oregano, and spices, and cook until the chicken becomes golden.
4. Pour the stock over and close the lid.
5. Cook on HIGH for 24 minutes.

6. Do a quick pressure release.
7. Open the lid and add the remaining ingredients.
8. Stir to combine and close the lid again.
9. Cook on HIGH for another 4 minutes.
10. Release the pressure quickly and serve drizzled with the sauce.
11. Enjoy!

Nutritional Values per serving:

Calories 455

Total Fats 26g

Carbs: 3g

Protein 55g

Dietary Fiber: 2g

Instant Pot Garlic Chicken

Prep Time: 8 Mins

TotalTime: 40 Mins

Serving: 4

Ingredients:

- 3 tbsp. coconut oil
- 5 cloves of garlic, minced
- 4 chicken breasts, halved
- Salt and pepper to taste
- 1 ½ cups water

Directions

1. Press the Sauté button on the Instant Pot and heat the coconut oil. Sauté the garlic until fragrant then stir in the chicken breasts. Season with salt and pepper to taste.
2. Stir for 5 minutes then pour in water.
3. Close the lid and seal off the vent. Press the Manual button and adjust the cooking time to 30 minutes.
4. Do natural pressure release.

Calories:591; Total Fat: 37.5g; Carbs: 1.1g; Dietary Fiber: 0.7g; Protein: 60.8g

Instant Pot Lemon Olive Chicken

Prep Time: 10 Mins

Total Time: 30 Mins

Serving: 4

Ingredients:

- 4 boneless skinless chicken breasts
- ½ cup coconut oil
- 1/4teaspoon black pepper
- 1/2teaspoon cumin
- 1teaspoon sea salt
- 1cup Homemade chicken bone-broth
- 2 tbsp. fresh lemon juice
- 1/2cup red onion, sliced
- 1can pitted green olives
- 1/2 lemon, thinly sliced

Direction

1. Generously season chicken breasts with cumin, pepper and salt; set your instant pot on sauté mode and melt coconut oil; add chicken and brown both sides.
2. Stir in the remaining ingredients; bring to a gentle simmer and then lock lid.
3. Cook on high for 10 minutes and then use quick release method to release pressure.

4. Serve and enjoy!

Nutritional Values per serving:

Calories 420

Total Fats 38.7g

Carbs: 0.6 g

Protein 42.4g

Dietary Fiber: 0.2g

Instant Pot Chicken Shawarma

Prep Time: 10 Mins

Total Time: 25 Mins

Serving: 8

Ingredients:

- 1 pound chicken thighs
- 1 pound chicken breasts, sliced
- 1/8 teaspoon cinnamon
- 1/4 teaspoon chili powder
- 1 teaspoon ground cumin
- 1/4 teaspoon ground allspice
- 1/4 teaspoon granulated garlic
- 1/2 teaspoon turmeric
- 1 teaspoon paprika
- Pinch of salt
- Pinch of pepper
- 1 cup Homemade chicken broth

Direction

1. Mix all ingredients in your instant pot and lock lid;
2. Cook on poultry setting for 15 minutes and the release pressure naturally.
3. Serve chicken with sauce over mashed sweet potato drizzled with tahini sauce.

Nutritional Values per serving:

Calories 223

Total Fats 8.7g

Carbs: 0.7 g

Protein 35.5g

Dietary Fiber: 0.2g

Italian-Inspired Creamy Chicken

Prep Time:5Mins

Cook Time:15Mins

Servings: 4

Ingredients:

- 4 boneless, skinless chicken thighs
- 1 teaspoon olive oil
- 1 cup homemade low-sodium chicken broth
- ⅓ cup unsweetened coconut cream or unsweetened almond cream
- 1½ Tablespoons arrowroot powder
- 1 Tablespoon organic basil pesto
- 1 Tablespoon organic Italian seasoning
- 2 Tablespoons organic minced garlic
- 1 Tablespoon organic minced onion
- Pinch of salt, pepper
- Fresh parsley

Direction

1. Press "Sauté" function on Instant Pot. Add olive oil.
2. Once hot, add onion, garlic. Cook 2 minutes. Add chicken. Cook 2 minutes per side, until golden brown. Season with salt, pepper, Italian seasoning. Stir in broth.

3. Lock, seal the lid. Press "Manual" button. Cook on HIGH 8 minutes.
4. When done, naturally release pressure 5 minutes, then quick release. Remove lid.
5. Press "Sauté" function. Stir in arrowroot powder. Stir to coat ingredients. Whisk in coconut cream, basil pesto. Stir. Allow to simmer until thickens. Season if needed.
6. Serve in bowls. Garnish with fresh parsley.

Calories: 242, Fat: 15g, Carbohydrates: 5.3g, Dietary Fiber: 1.8gg, Protein: 26g

Instant Pot Pesto Chicken

Prep Time: 10 Mins

TotalTime: 40 Mins

Serving: 4

Ingredients:

- 2 cups basil leaves
- ¼ cup extra virgin olive oil
- 5 sun-dried tomatoes
- Salt and pepper to taste
- 4 chicken breasts

Directions

1. Put in the food processor the basil leaves, olive oil, and tomatoes. Season with salt and people to taste. Add a cup of water if needed.
2. Place the chicken in the Instant Pot. Pour over the pesto sauce.
3. Close the lid and seal off the vent. Press the Manual button and adjust the cooking time to 30 minutes.

Do natural pressure release.

Calories:556; Total Fat: 32.7g; Carbs: 1.1g; Dietary Fiber: 0.7g; Protein:60.8g

Lemon Chicken

Prep Time:4 Mins

Cook Time: 15Mins

Servings: 3

Ingredients:

- 3 boneless, skinless chicken thighs or chicken breasts
- 1/2 small yellow onion, finely chopped
- 2 garlic cloves, minced
- 1 Tablespoons organic Italian seasoning
- 1/4 teaspoon organic smoked or regular paprika
- Zest and juice from 1 lemon
- 1/4 lemon, thinly sliced
- ½ cup homemade low-sodium chicken broth
- 1/4 Tablespoon fresh parsley, finely chopped
- 1 Tablespoons olive oil
- 1/2 Tablespoons ghee clarified butter
- 1/2 teaspoon organic garlic powder
- Pinch of salt, pepper

Direction

1. In a bowl, combine salt, pepper, garlic powder, paprika, Italian seasoning. Coat chicken on all sides with mixture.
2. Press "Sauté" function on Instant Pot. Add the olive oil.

3. Once hot, cook garlic, onions 2 minutes, stirring occasionally. Add chicken. Sear on all sides. Stir in ghee, lemon juice, lemon zest.
4. Place lemon slices on top of chicken.
5. Lock, seal lid. Press "Manual" button. Cook on HIGH 8 minutes.
6. When done, naturally release pressure 5 minutes, then quick release. Remove lid.
7. Serve on a platter. Garnish with fresh parsley, fresh lemon slices. Serve.

Calories: 380, Fat: 22.1g, Carbohydrates: 1.8g, Dietary Fiber: 0.5g, Protein: 42.5g

Delicious Beef Stew

Servings: 4

Cooking Time: 30 minutes

Ingredients:

- 2 ½ lbs chuck roast, boneless
- 1 cup chicken stock
- ½ cup balsamic vinegar
- 1 tbsp Worcestershire sauce
- 1 tbsp soy sauce
- 1 tbsp honey
- ½ tsp red pepper flakes
- 4 garlic cloves, chopped

Directions:

1. Add all ingredients into the instant pot and stir well.
2. Seal pot with lid and cook on high for 30 minutes.
3. Allow to release pressure naturally then open the lid.
4. Serve and enjoy.

Nutritional Values per serving:

Calories: 648; Carbohydrates: 7g; Protein: 94.3g; Fat: 23.7g; Sugar: 5.5g; Sodium: 647mg

Classic Lamb Leg

Servings: 4

Cooking Time: 15 minutes

Ingredients:

- 2 lbs leg of lamb, boneless and cut into chunks
- 2 tbsp tomato paste
- ½ cup beef stock
- 1 tsp oregano, chopped
- 2 tsp thyme, chopped
- 1 tsp rosemary, chopped
- 2 carrots, chopped
- 1 cup onion, chopped
- 1 cup red wine
- 4 garlic cloves, sliced
- 1 tbsp olive oil
- Pepper
- Salt

Directions:

1. Season meat with pepper and salt.
2. Add oil into the instant pot and set the pot on sauté mode.
3. Add meat to the pot and sauté until brown.
4. Add garlic and sauté for 30 seconds.

5. Add red wine and stir well.
6. Add remaining ingredients to the pot and stir well.
7. Seal pot with lid and cook on high for 15 minutes.
8. Allow to release pressure naturally then open the lid.
9. Serve and enjoy.

Nutritional Values per serving:

Calories: 542; Carbohydrates: 10.6g; Protein: 65.3g; Fat: 20.4g; Sugar: 4.2g; Sodium: 343mg

Asian Pork

Servings: 4

Cooking Time: 8 minutes

Ingredients:

- 1 ½ lbs pork shoulder, boneless and cut into strips
- 1 cup scallions, chopped
- 1 tbsp cornstarch
- 1 tbsp water
- 3 cups cabbage, sliced
- 2 garlic cloves, minced
- 1 tbsp sesame oil
- ¼ cup dry sherry
- ¼ cup soy sauce
- ½ cup chicken stock
- 0.5 oz dried mushrooms, cut into pieces

Directions:

1. Add meat into the instant pot along with garlic, oil, sherry, soy sauce, mushrooms, and stock. Stir well.
2. Seal pot with lid and cook on high for 8 minutes.
3. Allow to release pressure naturally then open the lid.
4. Add cabbage and stir well. Cook on sauté mode until cabbage is softened.

5. In a small bowl, mix together cornstarch and 1 tablespoon of water and pour into the pot. Stir until thickened, about 1-2 minutes.
6. Add scallions and stir well.
7. Serve and enjoy.

Nutritional Values per serving:

Calories: 568; Carbohydrates: 8.6g; Protein: 42g; Fat: 40g; Sugar: 2.7g; Sodium: 1124mg

Salsa Pork

Servings: 4

Cooking Time: 15 minutes

Ingredients:

- 2 lbs pork shoulder, boneless and cut into chunks
- ¼ cup fresh cilantro, chopped
- ½ cup chicken stock
- 1 tsp dried oregano
- 1 tsp ground cumin
- 1 tbsp honey
- oz can tomatoes, drained and diced
- 16 oz salsa
- Pepper
- Salt

Directions:

1. Season meat with pepper and salt.
2. Add meat, stock, oregano, cumin, honey, tomatoes, and salsa to the pot.
3. Seal pot with lid and cook on high for 15 minutes.
4. Allow to release pressure naturally then open the lid.
5. Shred the meat using a fork.
6. Add cilantro and stir well.
7. Serve and enjoy.

Nutritional Values per serving:

Calories: 735; Carbohydrates: 17.3g; Protein: 55.7g; Fat: 48.9g; Sugar: 11.4g; Sodium: 1189mg

BBQ Pork Ribs

Servings: 6

Cooking Time: 30 minutes

Ingredients:

- 1 cup water
- 3 lbs pork ribs
- ¼ cup tomato sauce
- 1 cup BBQ sauce
- ½ tsp black pepper
- ½ tsp dried oregano
- 1 tsp garlic powder
- 2 tsp paprika
- 1 tbsp brown sugar
- ½ tsp salt

Directions:

1. In a small bowl, mix together all spices.
2. In another bowl, mix together tomato sauce and ½ cup BBQ sauce.
3. Rub spice mixture over the pork ribs then toss ribs with sauce mixture.
4. Add pork ribs and water to the instant pot.
5. Seal pot with lid and cook on high for 30 minutes.

6. Release pressure using quick release method than open the lid.
7. Preheat the broiler. Place ribs on a baking tray and top with remaining BBQ sauce and broil for 3-5 minutes.
8. Serve and enjoy.

Nutritional Values per serving:

Calories: 694; Carbohydrates: 18.1g; Protein: 60.4g; Fat: 40.4g; Sugar: 12.9g; Sodium: 847mg

BBQ Pulled Pork

Servings: 4

Cooking Time: 15 minutes

Ingredients:

- 2 lbs pork shoulder, boneless and cut into chunks
- 1 cup beer
- 1 tbsp vinegar
- ¾ cup BBQ sauce
- 1/8 tsp cayenne pepper
- 1 tsp black pepper
- ¼ tsp oregano
- ½ tsp onion powder
- 1 tsp ground cumin
- 2 tsp chili powder
- 2 tsp paprika
- 1 tbsp brown sugar
- 1 tsp sea salt

Directions:

1. In a small bowl, mix together all the spice.
2. Add meat in a large bowl. Rub spice mixture all over the meat.
3. Pour vinegar and BBQ sauce over the meat and stir well.

4. Add beer and meat mixture into the instant pot.
5. Seal pot with lid and cook on high for 15 minutes.
6. Release pressure using quick release method than open the lid.
7. Shred the meat using a fork and serve.

Nutritional Values per serving:

Calories: 779; Carbohydrates: 23.5g; Protein: 53.6g; Fat: 49.2g; Sugar: 14.8g; Sodium: 1165mg

Pork Chops with Gravy

Servings: 4

Cooking Time: 18 minutes

Ingredients:

- 2 ½ lbs pork chops
- 1 tbsp cornstarch
- 2 tbsp water
- 1 cup chicken stock
- ½ tsp thyme
- 2 tbsp dried onion, minced
- 3 garlic cloves, smashed
- ¼ cup dry white wine
- 2 onions, sliced
- 2 tbsp olive oil
- Pepper
- Salt

Directions:

1. Season meat with pepper and salt and set aside.
2. Add oil into the instant pot and set the pot on sauté mode.
3. Add onion to the pot and sauté for 10 minutes.
4. Add garlic and wine and stir well.

5. Add thyme and dried onion. Add seasoned pork chops with stock. Stir well to combine.
6. Seal pot with lid and cook on high for 8 minutes.
7. Allow to release pressure naturally than open the lid.
8. Remove pork chops from pot and place on a plate.
9. In a small bowl, mix together cornstarch and water and pour into the instant pot and cook on sauté mode until gravy thickens.
10. Pour gravy over pork chops and serve.

Nutritional Values per serving:

Calories: 636; Carbohydrates: 3.9g; Protein: 88.7g; Fat: 26.1g; Sugar: 0.6g; Sodium: 390mg

Spicy & Smoky Beef

Servings: 4

Cooking Time: 15 minutes

Ingredients:

- 1 ¾ lbs flank steak, cut into strips
- ½ cup chicken stock
- ½ cup tomato sauce
- 1 onion, sliced
- 2 bell peppers, sliced
- ½ tsp oregano
- 1 tsp paprika
- 1 chipotle pepper in adobo sauce
- 3 garlic cloves, minced
- 2 tbsp olive oil
- Pepper
- Salt

Directions:

1. Season meat with pepper and salt.
2. Add oil into the instant pot and set the pot on sauté mode.
3. Add meat to the pot and sauté until brown.
4. Add remaining ingredients into the pot and stir well to combine.

5. Seal pot with lid and cook on high for 15 minutes.
6. Allow to release pressure naturally then open the lid.
7. Shred the meat using a fork and serve,

Nutritional Values per serving:

Calories: 492; Carbohydrates: 10.2g; Protein: 57.1g; Fat: 24.2g; Sugar: 5.6g; Sodium: 490mg

Coconut Beef Curry

Servings: 4

Cooking Time: 15 minutes

Ingredients:

- 1 ½ lbs beef, boneless and cut into chunks
- ½ cup basil, sliced
- 2 tbsp brown sugar
- 2 tbsp fish sauce
- ¼ cup chicken stock
- ¾ cup coconut milk
- 2 tbsp curry paste
- 1 onion, sliced
- 1 bell pepper, sliced
- 1 sweet potato, peeled and cut into chunks

Directions:

1. Add all ingredients except basil into the instant pot and stir well.
2. Seal pot with lid and cook on high for 15 minutes.
3. Allow to release pressure naturally then open the lid.
4. Add basil and stir well.
5. Serve over rice and enjoy.
6. Nutritional Values per serving:
7. Calories: 538; Carbohydrates: 20.2g; Protein: 54.8g; Fat: 25.9g; Sugar: 10.8g; Sodium: 875mg

Classic Sirloin Tips with Gravy

Servings: 4

Cooking Time: 10 minutes

Ingredients:

- 1 ½ lbs beef tips
- 1 tbsp cornstarch
- 2 tbsp water
- 1 cup chicken stock
- ¼ cup dry sherry
- 1 ½ tsp thyme
- 2 tbsp dried onion, minced
- 8 oz mushrooms, sliced
- 2 onions, sliced
- Pepper
- Salt

Directions:

1. In a small bowl, mix together cornstarch and water. Set aside
2. Season meat with pepper and salt.
3. Add meat to the pot along with remaining ingredients and stir well.
4. Seal pot with lid and cook on high for 10 minutes.
5. Allow to release pressure naturally then open the lid.

6. Remove meat from pot and place on a dish.
7. Add cornstarch mixture to the pot and cook on sauté mode until gravy thickens.
8. Return meat to the pot and stir well.
9. Serve and enjoy.

Nutritional Values per serving:

Calories: 426; Carbohydrates: 5.3g; Protein: 47.9g; Fat: 22.9g; Sugar: 1.7g; Sodium: 341mg

Moist & Tender Chuck Roast

Servings: 6

Cooking Time: 20 minutes

Ingredients:

- 3 lbs beef chuck roast, boneless and cut into chunks
- 2 tbsp parsley, chopped
- ½ cup red wine
- ½ cup chicken stock
- 1 tbsp soy sauce
- 2 tbsp tomato paste
- ½ tsp thyme
- 3 garlic cloves, crushed
- 2 celery ribs, chopped
- 2 carrots, peeled and sliced
- 2 onions, chopped
- Pepper
- Salt

Directions:

1. Season meat with pepper and salt and set aside.
2. Add onions, wine, stock, soy sauce, tomato paste, thyme, garlic, celery, carrots, pepper and salt to the pot and stir well. Place meat on top.
3. Seal pot with lid and cook on high for 20 minutes.

4. Allow to release pressure naturally then open the lid.
5. Shred the meat using a fork.
6. Add parsley and stir well.
7. Serve and enjoy.

Nutritional Values per serving:

Calories: 872; Carbohydrates: 7.9g; Protein: 60.5g; Fat: 63.3g; Sugar: 3.5g; Sodium: 409mg

Honey Pork Roast

Servings: 2

Cooking Time: 35 minutes

Ingredients:

- 1 lb pork roast
- 1 tbsp soy sauce
- 2 tbsp grated parmesan cheese
- ½ tbsp olive oil
- ½ tbsp garlic, minced
- ½ cup chicken stock
- ½ tbsp cornstarch
- ½ tbsp basil
- 2 tbsp honey
- Salt

Directions:

1. Add all ingredients into the instant pot and stir well.
2. Seal pot with lid and cook on meat mode for 35 minutes.
3. Allow to release pressure naturally than open the lid.
4. Stir well and serve warm.

Nutritional Values per serving:

Calories: 618; Carbohydrates: 20.6g; Protein: 68.5g; Fat: 27.3g; Sugar: 17.6g; Sodium: 968mg

Simple Meatballs

Servings: 2

Cooking Time: 25 minutes

Ingredients:

- 1 egg
- ¼ cup onion, chopped
- ¾ lb ground pork
- ¾ tsp brown sugar
- ¼ cup coconut milk
- 1 tbsp breadcrumbs

Directions:

1. **In a bowl, combine together meat, breadcrumbs, and egg.**
2. Make small balls from meat mixture.
3. Add coconut milk and prepared meatballs into the instant pot.
4. Add onion and brown sugar and stir well.
5. Seal pot with lid and cook on high for 25 minutes.
6. Allow to release pressure naturally then open the lid.
7. Serve warm and enjoy.

Nutritional Values per serving:

Calories: 367; Carbohydrates: 6.7g; Protein: 48.6g; Fat: 15.5g; Sugar: 3.1g; Sodium: 158mg

Shredded Thyme Pork

Servings: 3

Cooking Time: 40 minutes

Ingredients:

- 1 lb pork belly, cut into cubes
- 1 tsp thyme
- 1 ½ tsp black pepper
- ½ cup onion, chopped
- ½ cup chicken stock
- 3 tbsp water
- 1 tbsp cornstarch
- ¼ tsp salt

Directions:

1. In a small bowl, mix together cornstarch and water and set aside.
2. Add remaining ingredients to the instant pot and stir well.
3. Seal pot with lid and cook on high for 35 minutes.
4. Release pressure using quick release method than open the lid.
5. Pour cornstarch mixture into the instant pot and stir well.
6. Serve and enjoy.

Nutritional Values per serving:

Calories: 654; Carbohydrates: 7.2g; Protein: 19.6g; Fat: 60.2g; Sugar: 1g; Sodium: 1324mg

Pineapple Cinnamon Pork

Servings: 2

Cooking Time: 25 minutes

Ingredients:

- ½ lb pork tenderloin, sliced
- ½ cup tomato puree
- ½ tsp rosemary
- ¼ cup onion, chopped
- 2 cloves
- ½ tsp cinnamon
- ½ tsp nutmeg
- ½ cup pineapple, cut into chunks
- 1 cup pineapple juice

Directions:

1. Add all ingredients except pineapple into the instant pot and stir well.
2. Seal pot with lid and cook on high for 25 minutes.
3. Release pressure using quick release method than open the lid.
4. Add pineapple chunks and stir well.
5. Serve and enjoy.

Nutritional Values per serving:

Calories: 284; Carbohydrates: 29.4g; Protein: 31.6g; Fat: 4.6g; Sugar: 20.3g; Sodium: 86mg

Spicy Celery Cauliflower Pork

Servings: 4

Cooking Time: 20 minutes

Ingredients:

- 2 lbs pork ribs, cut into pieces
- 1 bay leaf
- ½ tsp red pepper flakes
- 1 tsp chili powder
- 3 tbsp olive oil
- 4 cups chicken stock
- ¼ cup parsley, chopped
- 1 cup cauliflower florets
- 1 cup celery, chopped
- 1 onion, chopped
- 1 leek chopped
- 1 tsp salt

Directions:

1. Add oil into the instant pot and set the pot on sauté mode.
2. Add meat to the pot and cook until brown. Remove meat from pot and set aside.
3. Add celery, onion, and salt and sauté for 4-5 minutes.

4. Return meat to the pot with remaining ingredients and stir well.
5. Seal pot with lid and cook on high for 20 minutes.
6. Allow to release pressure naturally then open the lid.
7. Serve and enjoy.

Nutritional Values per serving:

Calories: 744; Carbohydrates: 6.1g; Protein: 62g; Fat: 51.5g; Sugar: 2.9g; Sodium: 1514mg

Delicious Curried Pork

Servings: 4

Cooking Time: 11 minutes

Ingredients:

- 1 lb pork, cut into strips
- 2 tsp curry powder
- 1 tsp fresh ginger, grated
- 2 tsp sesame oil
- 1 tbsp rice vinegar
- 1 spring onion, chopped
- 1 garlic clove, crushed
- 1 medium onion, sliced
- ¼ cup olive oil
- ½ tsp salt

Directions:

1. Add olive oil into the instant pot and set the pot on sauté mode.
2. Add meat into the pot and cook on sauté mode for 5 minutes. Remove meat from pot and set aside.
3. Add onion, spring onion, and garlic and sauté for 3-4 minutes.

4. Add ginger and curry powder. Add salt and stir well and cook for 2 minutes more.
5. Drizzle with sesame oil and serve.

Nutritional Values per serving:

Calories: 311; Carbohydrates: 4g; Protein: 30.3g; Fat: 19.1g; Sugar: 1.3g; Sodium: 358mg

Asian Pork with gravy

Servings: 2

Cooking Time: 15 minutes

Ingredients:

- 10 oz pork, boneless and cut into strips
- 1 tsp pepper
- 3 tbsp sesame oil
- 2 tbsp oyster sauce
- 2 tbsp fish sauce
- 2 garlic cloves
- 1 cup mushrooms, chopped
- 2 spring onion, chopped
- 1 small onion, chopped
- ½ tsp salt

Directions:

1. Add oil into the pot and set the pot on sauté mode.
2. Add garlic, onion, and meat and sauté for 1-2 minutes.
3. Add spring onion and sauté for 2-3 minutes.
4. Add mushrooms and stir well.
5. Add oyster sauce and fish sauce. Stir well and cook for 2-3 minutes.

6. Season with pepper. Add ¼ cup of water and simmer for 10 minutes.
7. Serve and enjoy.

Nutritional Values per serving:

Calories: 425; Carbohydrates: 8.3g; Protein: 40.1g; Fat: 25.6g; Sugar: 3.1g; Sodium: 2168mg

Apple and Cherry Sweetened Pork Tenderloin

Preparation Time: 55 minutes

Serving: 4

Nutritional Values per serving: Calories 349; Carbs 18g; Fat 12g; Protein 40g

Ingredients

- 1 ¼ pounds Pork Tenderloin
- 1 chopped Celery Stalk
- 2 cups Apples, peeled and chopped
- 1 cup Cherries, pitted
- ½ cup Apple Juice
- ½ cup Water
- ¼ cup Onions, chopped
- Salt and Pepper, to taste
- 2 tbsp Olive Oil

Directions

1. Heat oil on SAUTÉ mode at High, and cook the onion and celery for 5 minutes until softened. Season the pork with salt and pepper, and add to the cooker. Brown for 2-3 minutes per side.
2. Then, top with apples and cherries, and pour the water and apple juice. Seal the lid and cook on MEAT/STEW mode for 40 minutes, at High pressure. Do a quick pressure release.

3. Slice the pork tenderloin and arrange on a platter. Spoon the apple-cheery sauce over the pork slices, to serve.

Pork Sausage with Cauliflower and Tater Tots

Preparation Time: 20 minutes

Serving: 6

Nutritional Values per serving: Calories 431; Carbs 66g; Fat 12g; Protein 23g

Ingredients

- 1 pound Pork Sausage, sliced
- 1 pound Tater Tots
- 1 pound Cauliflower Florets, frozen and thawed
- 10 ounces canned Mushroom Soup
- 10 ounces canned Cauliflower Soup
- 10 ounces Evaporated Milk
- Salt and Pepper, to taste

Directions

1. Place roughly ¼ of the sausage slices in your pressure cooker. In a bowl, whisk together the soups and milk. Pour some of the mixtures over the sausages.
2. Top the sausage slices with ¼ of the cauliflower florets followed by ¼ of the tater tots. Pour some of the soup mixtures again. Repeat the layers until you use up all ingredients. Seal the lid, and cook on PRESSURE COOK/MANUAL for 10 minutes, at High. When ready, do a quick release.

Spicy Ground Pork with Peas

Preparation Time: 55 minutes

Serving: 6

Nutritional Values per serving: Calories 510; Carbs 4g; Fat 34g; Protein 41g

Ingredients

- 2 pounds Ground Pork
- 1 Onion, diced
- 1 can diced Tomatoes
- 1 can Peas
- 5 Garlic Cloves, crushed
- 3 tbsp Butter
- 1 Serrano Pepper, chopped
- 1 cup Beef Broth
- 1 tsp ground Ginger
- 2 tsp ground Coriander
- 1 tsp Salt
- ¾ tsp Cumin
- ¼ tsp Cayenne Pepper
- ½ tsp Turmeric
- ½ tsp Black Pepper

Directions

1. Melt butter on SAUTÉ at High. Add onions and cook for 3 minutes, until soft. Stir in the spices and garlic and cook for 2 more minutes. Add pork and cook until browned. ADD broth, serrano pepper, peas, and tomatoes. Seal the lid and cook for 30 minutes on MEAT/STEW at High. Release the pressure naturally for 10 minutes.

Tamari Sauce Pork Belly with Garlic

Preparation Time: 40 minutes

Serving: 6

Nutritional Values per serving: Calories 520; Carbs 5g; Fat 28g; Protein 49g

Ingredients

- 4 Garlic Cloves, sliced
- ½ tsp ground Cloves
- 1 tsp grated fresh Ginger
- 1 ½ pounds Pork Belly, sliced
- 2 ¼ cups Water
- ¼ cup White Wine
- ½ cup Yellow Onions, peeled and chopped
- ¼ cup Tamari Sauce
- 1 tsp Sugar Maple Syrup
- 4 cups short-grain White Rice, cooked, warm

Directions

1. Brown pork belly, for about 6 minutes per side, on SAUTÉ at High. Add the remaining ingredients. Seal the lid and cook for 25 minutes on BEANS/CHILI at High Pressure. Cook until the meat is tender.
2. Once ready, switch the pressure release valve to open, and do a quick pressure release. Serve with rice.

Braised Chili Pork Chops

Preparation Time: 30 minutes

Serving: 4

Nutritional Values per serving: Calories 437; Carbs 11g; Fat 24g; Protein 44g

Ingredients

4 Pork Chops

1 Onion, chopped

2 tbsp Chili Powder

14 ounces canned Tomatoes with Green Chilies

1 Garlic Clove, minced

½ cup Beer

½ cup Vegetable Stock

1 tsp Olive Oil

- Salt and Pepper, to taste

Directions

1. Heat oil on SAUTÉ mode at High. Add onion, garlic, and chili powder and cook for 2 minutes. Add the pork chops and cook until browned on all sides. Stir in the tomatoes, broth, and beer. Season with salt and pepper.
2. Seal the lid and cook for 20 minutes on PRESSURE COOK/MANUAL at High. Quick release the pressure.

Delicious Short Ribs with Mango Sauce

Preparation Time: 35 minutes

Serving: 6

Nutritional Values per serving: Calories 625; Carbs 41g; Fat 31g; Protein 62g

Ingredients

- 1 lb Short Ribs, cut into 3-inch pieces
- 18 ounces canned Mango, undrained
- ½ tsp Black Pepper, to taste
- ½ tsp ground Parsley
- 1 tsp Salt
- 1 cup Onions, sliced
- 1-inch piece Ginger, finely chopped
- ½ tsp Garlic, minced
- ½ cup Tomato Paste
- 3 tsp Olive Oil
- ½ cup Soy sauce
- 2 tbsp Vinegar
- ¼ cup prepared Arrowroot slurry

Directions

1. On SAUTÉ, heat oil and cook the onions until tender, about 4 minutes. Stir in the remaining ingredients, except the arrowroot. Seal the lid, press PRESSURE

COOK/MANUAL and cook for 20 minutes at High. Once ready, do a quick release. Stir in the arrowroot slurry and cook on SAUTÉ at High until the sauce thickens.

Classy Pork Ribs in Walnut Sauce

Preparation Time: 30 minutes

Serving: 4

Nutritional Values per serving: Calories 273; Carbs 4g; Fat 16g; Protein 27g

Ingredients

- 1 pound Pork Ribs
- ¼ cup Roasted Walnuts, chopped
- 4 Garlic Cloves, minced
- 1 ½ cups Beef Broth
- 2 tbsp Apple Cider Vinegar
- 3 tbsp Butter
- ½ tsp Red Pepper Flakes
- 1 tsp Sage
- Salt and Black Pepper, to taste

Directions

1. Melt butter on SAUTÉ at High. Season the ribs with salt, pepper, sage, and pepper flakes. Place them in the pressure cooker and brown, for about 5 minutes. Stir in the remaining ingredients. Seal the lid.
2. Cook for 20 minutes on PRESSURE COOK/MANUAL at High. Release the pressure quickly. Serve drizzled with the sauce.

Succulent Short Ribs with Red Wine Gravy

Preparation Time: 70 minutes

Serving: 4

Nutritional Values per serving: Calories 479; Carbs 4g; Fat 31g; Protein 46

Ingredients

- 2 pounds boneless Beef Short Ribs, cut into 3-inch pieces
- 1 tsp Kosher Salt
- ½ tsp ground Black Pepper
- ½ Onion, chopped
- ½ cup Red Wine
- 3 tbsp Oil
- ½ tbsp Tomato paste
- 2 Carrots, sliced

Directions

1. Rub the ribs on all sides with salt, and black pepper. Heat the oil on SAUTÉ at High, and brown short ribs on all sides, 3-5 minutes per side, working in batches. Remove ribs to a plate.
2. Add onions and cook for 3-5 minutes, until tender. Pour in wine and tomato paste to deglaze by scraping any browned bits from the bottom of the cooker. Cook for 2 minutes until wine has reduced slightly.

3. Return ribs to pot and cover with carrots, garlic, parsley, rosemary, and oregano. Pour beef broth over ribs and vegetables. Hit Cancel to stop SAUTÉ mode at High. Seal the lid, and select MEAT/STEW at High Pressure for 35 minutes. When ready, let pressure release naturally for 10 minutes. Transfer ribs to a plate.
4. Remove and discard vegetables and herbs. Stir in mushrooms. Press SAUTÉ at High and cook until mushrooms are soft, 2-4 minutes. In a bowl, add water and cornstarch and mix until smooth.
5. Pour this slurry into broth, stirring constantly, until it thickens slightly, 2 minutes. Season gravy with salt and pepper to taste. Pour over the ribs and garnish with minced parsley to serve.

Tangy Pork Shoulder with Tomato Sauce

Preparation Time: 35 minutes

Serving: 6

Nutritional Values per serving: Calories 503; Carbs 11g; Fat 41g; Protein 32g

Ingredients

- 1 ½ pounds Pork Shoulder, cubed
- 1 cup Tomato Sauce
- ½ cups Buttermilk
- 1 cup Green Onions, chopped
- 2 tsp Butter, melted
- ¼ tsp Chili Pepper
- 3 Garlic Cloves, minced
- ½ tbsp Cilantro
- Salt and Black Pepper, to taste

Directions

1. Select SAUTÉ at High and melt butter. Cook onions and minced garlic until soft, 2-3 minutes. Add the remaining ingredients, except for the buttermilk. Sea the lid and cook for 25 minutes on MEAT/STEW at High.
2. Once cooking is complete, do a quick pressure release. Stir in the sour cream until well incorporated.

Yummy Pork Loin Chops with Sauerkraut

Preparation Time: 35 minutes

Serving: 4

Nutritional Values per serving: Calories 383; Carbs 11g; Fat 18g; Protein 22g

Ingredients

- 4 Pork Loin Chops, boneless
- 4 cups Sauerkraut, shredded
- 1 cup dry White Wine
- cloves Garlic, peeled and crushed
- 1 cup Carrots, coarsely chopped
- ½ cup Celery, coarsely chopped
- 2 Onions, sliced
- 2 cups Vegetable Stock
- 2 tsp Mustard
- 1 tsp Salt
- ½ tsp Chili powder
- ½ cup Tomato Paste
- ½ tsp ground Black Pepper

Directions

1. Place the pork on the bottom of the pressure cooker. Add the shredded cabbage on top of the pork. Add in the remaining ingredients and seal the lid. Select

BEANS/CHILI and cook for 30 minutes at High Pressure. Once cooking is done, do a quick pressure release. Serve immediately.

Sloppy Joes and Coleslaw

Preparation Time: 30 minutes

Serving: 6

Nutritional Values per serving: Calories 313; Carbs 18g; Fat 22g; Protein 24g

Ingredients

- 1 cup Tomatoes, chopped
- 1 Onion, chopped
- 1 Carrot, chopped
- 1 pound Ground Beef
- 1 Bell Pepper, chopped
- ½ cup Rolled Oats
- 4 tbsp Apple Cider Vinegar
- 1 tbsp Olive Oil
- 4 tbsp Tomato Paste
- 1 cup Water
- 2 tsp Garlic Powder
- 1 tbsp Worcestershire Sauce
- 1 ½ tsp Salt
- Coleslaw:
- ½ Red Onion, chopped
- 1 tbsp Honey
- ½ head Cabbage, sliced
- 2 Carrots, grated

- 2 tbsp Apple Cider Vinegar
- 1 tbsp Dijon Mustard

Directions

1. Warm olive oil on SAUTÉ at High, and brown the meat for 3-4 minutes. Sauté onions, carrots, pepper, garlic, and salt, until soft. Stir in tomatoes, vinegar, Worcestershire sauce, water, and paste.
2. When starting to boil, stir in the oats. Seal the lid, select BEANS/CHILI for 25 minutes at High. Do a quick pressure release. Mix all slaw ingredients in a large bowl. Serve the sloppy joes with the slaw.

Savory Fettuccine with Beef Sausage

Preparation Time: 40 minutes

Serving: 6

Nutritional Values per serving: Calories 512; Carbs 58g; Fat 10g; Protein 23g

Ingredients

- 1 pound Beef Sausage, chopped
- 1 pound dried Fettuccine Pasta
- ½ cup dry White Wine
- 1 clove Garlic, minced
- ½ cups Green Peas, frozen
- ½ Chipotle Pepper, seeded and chopped
- 1 cup Black Beans, soaked overnight
- 2 Yellow Bell Peppers, seeded and chopped
- 2 tsp Olive Oil
- 2 cups Water
- 1 cup Scallions, chopped
- 1 (28 ounce can whole plum Tomatoes
- ¼ tsp crushed Red Pepper flakes
- 1 cup Parmesan cheese, shredded
- ½ tsp dried Basil
- ½ tsp dried Oregano
- 1 tsp Salt
- ¼ tsp ground Black Pepper

- Fresh Parsley, for garnish

Directions

1. Heat the oil, and sauté the scallions, peppers, and garlic for 3 minutes on SAUTÉ mode at High. Stir in the beef sausage. Sear until lightly browned, for about 3-4 minutes.
2. Add the remaining ingredients, except for the parsley and parmesan cheese. Add more water if needed. Seal the lid, Select PRESSURE COOK/MANUAL mode and cook for 10 more minutes at High Pressure. Once ready, do a quick release. Stir in parmesan cheese until melted. Serve sprinkled with parsley.

Luscious Italian Sausage over Muffins

Preparation Time: 20 minutes

Serving: 8

Nutritional Values per serving: Calories 478; Carbs 29g; Fat 31g; Protein 28g

Ingredients

- 8 toasted English Muffins, split
- 1 ½ pounds Italian Sausage
- 1 ¼ cups Milk
- ¼ cup Flour
- 1 cup Eggplants, sliced
- 1 cup Bone Broth
- 1 tsp Salt
- ½ tsp Black Pepper, freshly cracked
- 2 sprigs dry Thyme
- 2 sprigs dry Rosemary

Directions

1. Select SAUTÉ at High and add in the eggplants and sausage. Cook for 5 minutes. Sprinkle with rosemary and thyme, and pour in the broth. Seal the lid, select on PRESSURE COOK/MANUAL and cook for 5 minutes at High.
2. Do quick pressure release. In a measuring cup, whisk flour and milk, and season with salt and pepper. Add

the mixture to the pressure cooker. Select SAUTÉ, and let simmer for 3 minutes, lid off. Spoon gravy over the toasted split muffins and enjoy.

Cheesy Rigatoni with Pancetta

Preparation Time: 30 minutes

Serving: 6

Nutritional Values per serving: Calories 481; Carbs 2g; Fat 32g; Protein 19g

Ingredients

- 1 ½ box Penne Pasta
- 6 slices Pancetta, fried and crumbled
- ½ cup Grana Padano cheese, grated
- 1 cup Cottage cheese
- 3 tsp Olive Oil
- 1 cup Yellow Onions, finely chopped
- 3 Garlic Cloves, finely minced
- 3 ½ cups Vegetable Broth
- 1 ½ cups Water
- 2 sprigs dry Rosemary
- Salt and freshly ground Black Pepper, to taste

Directions

1. Add rigatoni, broth, water, salt, black pepper, and rosemary to your pressure cooker. Seal the lid, select PRESSURE COOK/MANUAL for 12 minutes at High Pressure. Once ready, do a quick pressure release. Set aside.

2. Select SAUTÉ at High and melt the butter. Cook onions and garlic, until fragrant, about 2-3 minutes. Add pancetta, cottage cheese, and rigatoni mixture back to the cooker, and toss until everything is well mixed.
3. Serve immediately topped with freshly grated Grana Padano cheese.

Delicious Pork Shoulder with White Cabbage

Preparation Time: 25 minutes

Serving: 6

Nutritional Values per serving: Calories 203; Carbs 13g; Fat 2g; Protein 25g

Ingredients

- 1 head Cabbage, shredded
- ½ cup Vegetable Stock
- 4 Cloves Garlic, finely minced
- 2 Red Onions, chopped
- 1 cup Tomato Puree
- 3 Tomatoes, chopped
- 1 ¼ pounds Pork Shoulder, boneless, cut into cubes
- 1 Bay Leaf
- ½ tsp Paprika, crushed
- Salt and Black Pepper, to taste

Directions

1. Select SAUTÉ at High and add the pork, onions and garlic. Cook the pork until lightly browned. Remove any fat. Add in the remaining ingredients. Seal the lid, press on PRESSURE COOK/MANUAL and cook for 15 minutes at High. Once cooking is complete, do a quick pressure release. Discard the bay leaf and serve.

Chuck Roast with Potatoes to Die for

Preparation Time: 50 minutes

Serving: 6

Nutritional Values per serving: Calories 441; Carbs 20g; Fat 17g; Protein 53g

Ingredients

- 2 ½ pounds Chuck Roast
- 1 pound Red Potatoes, chopped
- 2 Carrots, chopped
- ½ cup Parsnip, chopped
- 1 cup Onions, sliced
- ½ cup Red Wine
- ½ Celery Stalk, sliced
- 1 tbsp Rosemary
- 1 tsp Thyme
- ½ tsp Pepper
- ½ tsp Salt
- 2 tbsp Tomato Paste
- 1 tbsp Garlic, minced
- 1 cup Beef Broth

Directions

1. Coat the cooker with cooking spray. In a bowl, combine the thyme, rosemary, salt, and pepper and rub the

mixture onto the meat. Place the meat inside the cooker and sear on all sides.

2. Add the remaining ingredients and seal the lid. Set to MEAT/STEW for 40 minutes at High. Once the cooking is over, do a quick pressure release. Serve and enjoy!

Ground Beef with Sauerkraut

Preparation Time: 25 minutes

Serving: 6

Nutritional Values per serving: Calories 337; Carbs 8g; Fat 20g; Protein 30g

Ingredients

- 1 ½ pounds Ground Beef
- 10 ounces canned Tomato Soup
- ½ cup Beef Broth
- 3 cups Sauerkraut
- 1 cup sliced Leeks
- 1 tbsp Butter
- 1 tsp Mustard Powder
- Salt and Pepper, to taste

Directions

1. Melt butter on SAUTÉ at High. Add leeks and cook for a few minutes, until soft. Add beef and brown, for a few minutes. Stir in the sauerkraut, broth and mustard powder and season with salt and pepper.
2. Seal the lid and cook for 20 minutes on SOUP/BROTH mode at High. When ready, do a quick pressure release.

Tempting Citrusy Beef

Preparation Time: 90 minutes

Serving: 6

Nutritional Values per serving: Calories 477; Carbs 8g; Fat 36g; Protein 35g

Ingredients

- Juice of 1 Lemon
- Juice of 2 Oranges
- 2 pounds Beef, cut into chunks
- 1 tbsp Butter
- 1 tbsp Italian Seasoning
- ½ tsp Sea Salt

Directions

1. Place the beef in the pressure cooker and sprinkle with salt, pepper, and seasoning. Massage the meat with hands to season it well. Pour the lemon and orange juice over and seal the lid.
2. Select PRESSURE COOK/MANUAL for 50 minutes, at High pressure. When the timer goes off, do a quick pressure release. Shred the meat inside the pot with two forks. Set to SAUTÉ mode at High, lid off.
3. Stir to combine well and cook for about 20 minutes, or until the liquid is absorbed. Add butter, give it a good stir, and cook for an additional 5 minutes.

Beef Ribs with Button Mushrooms

Preparation Time: 30 minutes

Serving: 6

Nutritional Values per serving: Calories 509; Carbs 9g; Fat 43g; Protein 22g

Ingredients

- 1 ½ pounds Beef Ribs
- 2 cups White Button Mushrooms, quartered
- 1 Onion, chopped
- ¼ cup Ketchup
- 2 cups Veggie Stock
- 1 cup chopped Carrots
- ¼ cup Olive Oil
- 1 tsp Garlic, minced
- Salt and Pepper, to taste

Directions

1. Heat the oil on SAUTÉ mode at High. Season the ribs with salt and pepper, and brown them on all sides. Then, set aside. Add the onion, garlic, carrots, and mushrooms and cook for 5 minutes.
2. Add the ribs back to the cooker and stir in the remaining ingredients. Seal the lid and cook for 35 minutes on MEAT/STEW at High pressure. When cooking is over, do a quick release.

Beef Medley with Blue Cheese

Preparation Time: 50 minutes

Serving: 6

Nutritional Values per serving: Calories 267; Carbs 6g; Fat 13g; Protein 30

Ingredients

- 1 pound Sirloin Steak, cut into cubes
- 6 ounces Blue Cheese, crumbled
- ½ Cabbage, diced
- 1 cup Parsnip, chopped
- 2 Red Bell Peppers, chopped
- 1 cup Beef Broth
- 2 cups canned Tomatoes, undrained
- 1 Onion, diced
- 1 tsp Garlic, minced
- Salt and Black Pepper, to taste
- Cooking spray, for greasing

Directions

1. Coat the cooker with cooking spray and add the sirloin steak. On SAUTÉ at High, brown the steak on all sides, for a few minutes. Then, add the remaining ingredients, except for the cheese.

2. Seal the lid and cook for 40 minutes on MEAT/STEW mode at High. Once cooking is complete, release the pressure quickly. Top with blue cheese, to serve.

Steak and Veggies with Ale Sauce

Preparation Time: 50 minutes

Serving: 6

Nutritional Values per serving: Calories 370; Carbs 32g; Fat 11g; Protein 36g

Ingredients

- 2 pounds Beef Steak, cut into 6 or 8 equal pieces
- 1 Sweet Onion, chopped
- 1 cup Celery, chopped
- 1 pound Sweet Potatoes, diced
- 2 Carrots, chopped
- 3 Garlic Cloves, minced
- 2 Bell Peppers, chopped
- 1 ½ cups Tomato Puree
- 1 cup Ale
- 1 Chicken Bouillon Cube
- Salt and Pepper, to taste
- 1 tbsp Olive Oil

Directions

1. Heat oil on SAUTÉ at High and sear the steaks, for a few minutes. Then, set aside. Press CANCEL. Arrange the veggies in the pressure cooker and top with the steak. In a bowl, whisk together bouillon cube, ale, and tomato puree. Pour over the steaks. Season with salt

and pepper, and seal the lid. Cook for 30 minutes on MEAT/STEW at High. Quick-release the pressure.

Beef Roast with Creamy Sour Sauce

Preparation Time: 35 minutes

Serving: 6

Nutritional Values per serving: Calories 340; Carbs 10g; Fat 19g; Protein 33g

Ingredients

- 1 ½ pounds Beef Roast, cubed
- 1 cup Onion, diced
- 1 can Cream of Mushroom Soup
- 1 ½ cups Sour Cream
- ½ cups Water
- ½ tbsp Cumin
- ½ tbsp Coriander
- 1 tbsp Garlic, minced
- 1 tbsp Butter
- ½ tsp Chili Powder
- Salt and Pepper, to taste

Directions

1. Melt butter on SAUTÉ at High and stir in the onion. Stir-fry until soft, for about 3 minutes. Add garlic and cook for one more minute. Add beef and cook until browned, for about 3 – 5 minutes.
2. Combine the remaining ingredients in a bowl and pour this mixture over the beef. Seal the lid and cook for 25

minutes on MEAT/STEW mode at High. Once done, do a quick release.

Corned Beef with Celery Sauce

Preparation Time: 50 minutes

Serving: 6

Nutritional Values per serving: Calories 287; Carbs 8g; Fat 20g; Protein 18g

Ingredients

- 1 ½ pounds Corned Beef Brisket
- 2 cups Cream of Celery Soup
- 1 tsp Garlic, minced
- 1 Onion, diced
- 1 cup Water
- 2 Tomatoes, diced
- 2 tsp Olive Oil
- Salt and Black Pepper, to taste

Directions

1. Season the beef with salt, and black pepper. Heat oil on SAUTÉ, and stir onions. Cook for 2 minutes, until translucent. Add garlic and cook for 1 minute.Add beef and sear on all sides, for a few minutes.
2. Pour in soup and water. Seal the lid, cook for 40 minutes on MEAT/STEW at High. Do a quick pressure release.

Beer-Dijon Braised Steak

Preparation Time: 40 minutes

Serving: 4

Nutritional Values per serving: Calories 525; Carbs 12g; Fat 21g; Protein 69g

Ingredients

- 4 Beef Steaks
- 12 ounces Dark Beer
- 2 tbsp Dijon Mustard
- 2 Carrots, chopped
- 1 tbsp Tomato Paste
- 1 Onion, chopped
- 1 tsp Paprika
- 2 tbsp Flour
- 1 cup Beef Broth
- Salt and Pepper, to taste
- Olive oil, to grease

Directions

1. Brush the meat with the mustard and season with paprika, salt, and pepper. Coat the pressure cooker with cooking spray and sear the steak on SAUTÉ mode at High. Remove steaks to a plate.
2. Press CANCEL. Pour ¼ cup water and scrape the bottom of the cooker. Wipe clean. Whisk in the tomato

paste and flour. Gradually stir in the remaining ingredients, except for the beer.

3. Return the steak to the cooker, pour in beer and seal the lid. Cook for 25 minutes on MEAT/STEW mode at High. When ready, release the pressure quickly and serve hot.

Tender Onion Beef Roast

Preparation Time: 55 minutes

Serving: 8

Nutritional Values per serving: Calories 369; Carbs 9g; Fat 16g; Protein 47g

Ingredients

- 3 pounds Beef Roast
- 2 Large Sweet Onions, sliced
- 1 envelope Onion Mix
- 1 cup Beef Broth
- 1 cup Tomato Juice
- 1 tsp Garlic, minced
- 2 tbsp Worcestershire Sauce
- 1 tbsp Olive Oil
- Salt and Pepper, to taste

Directions

1. Warm the oil on SAUTÉ mode at High. Season the beef with salt and pepper, and sear on all sides. Transfer to a plate. Add onions, and cook for 3 minutes. Stir in garlic and cook for 1 minute.
2. Add the beef and stir in the remaining ingredients. Seal the lid and cook for 40 minutes on MEAT/STEW at High. Release the pressure naturally, for 10 minutes.

Holiday Pork Ham Hock

Preparation Time: 55 minutes

Servings 6

Nutritional Values per serving: 304 Calories; 19.1g Fat; 2.6g Carbs; 30.5g Protein; 0.6g Sugars

Ingredients

- 1 cup water
- 1/2 cup ale beer
- Sea salt and ground black pepper, to taste
- 1/2 teaspoon cayenne pepper, or more to taste
- 1/2 teaspoon marjoram
- 1/2 teaspoon dried sage, crushed
- A bunch of scallions, chopped
- 2 pounds pork ham hocks
- 2 bay leaves
- 2 garlic cloves, minced

Directions

1. Place all of the above ingredients in the Instant Pot.
2. Secure the lid. Choose the "Meat/Stew" setting and cook at High pressure for 45 minutes. Once cooking is complete, use a natural pressure release; carefully remove the lid.

3. Remove ham hocks from the Instant Pot; allow them to cool enough to be handled. Remove meat from ham hocks and return it to the cooking liquid.
4. Serve on individual plates and enjoy!

Old-Fashioned Pork Stew

Preparation Time: 50 minutes

Servings 6

Nutritional Values per serving: 307 Calories; 17.2g Fat; 4.8g Carbs; 31.1g Protein; 2.5g Sugars

Ingredients

- 1 ½ tablespoons lard, at room temperature
- 1 ½ pounds pork stew meat, cubed
- Hickory smoked salt and ground black pepper, to taste
- 1 cup leeks, chopped
- 2 garlic cloves, minced
- 1 (1-inch piece fresh ginger root, grated
- 1 teaspoon mustard seeds
- 1 teaspoon fennel seeds
- 2 tablespoons soy sauce
- 1/4 cup dry red wine
- 5 cups beef bone broth
- 1/4 cup fresh parsley leaves, roughly chopped

Directions

1. Press the "Sauté" button and melt the lard. Now, brown pork stew meat for 4 to 6 minutes, stirring occasionally.

2. Season the pork with salt and black pepper to taste and set it aside. In pan drippings, cook the leeks along with garlic and ginger until tender and aromatic.
3. Add the pork back to the Instant Pot; add the remaining ingredients and gently stir to combine. Secure the lid.
4. Choose "Meat/Stew" mode and cook at High pressure for 40 minutes. Once cooking is complete, use a quick release; remove the lid carefully.
5. Ladle into individual bowls and serve garnished with fresh parsley leaves. Bon appétit!

Mexican-Style Meatballs

Preparation Time: 15 minutes

Servings 6

Nutritional Values per serving: 476 Calories; 24.5g Fat; 33.2g Carbs; 27.9g Protein; 19.5g Sugars

Ingredients

- 1 pound ground pork
- 2 slices bacon, chopped
- 1 white onion, minced
- 1 teaspoon garlic, minced
- 1/3 cup tortilla chips, crushed
- 1/2 cup Romano cheese, freshly grated
- 1 egg
- Sea salt and ground black pepper, to taste
- 1 teaspoon dried marjoram
- 1 cup ketchup
- 2 cups tomato sauce
- 2 chipotle chile in adobo
- 2 tablespoons fresh cilantro

Directions

1. Thoroughly combine ground pork, bacon, onion, garlic, tortilla chips, Romano cheese, egg, salt, black pepper, and marjoram. Shape the mixture into balls.

2. Now, add ketchup, tomato sauce, and chipotle chile in adobo to the Instant Pot. Place the meatballs in your Instant Pot.
3. Secure the lid. Choose the "Manual" setting and cook at High pressure for 6 minutes. Once cooking is complete, use a quick pressure release; carefully remove the lid.
4. Serve warm garnished with fresh cilantro. Enjoy!

Easy Pork Soup with Corn

Preparation Time: 15 minutes

Servings 4

Nutritional Values per serving: 358 Calories; 9.1g Fat; 32.4g Carbs; 36.1g Protein; 0.8g Sugars

Ingredients

- 1 tablespoon olive oil
- 1/2 cup onion, chopped
- 1 pound pork stew meat, cubed
- 4 cups water
- 1/4 teaspoon bay leaf, ground
- 1/2 teaspoon dried basil
- 1 teaspoon celery seeds
- 1 cup corn, torn into pieces

Directions

1. Press the "Sauté" button to preheat your Instant Pot. Heat the olive oil; cook the onion until tender and translucent.
2. Add pork and continue to cook until it is delicately browned. Add water, ground bay leaf, basil, and celery seeds to the Instant Pot.

3. Secure the lid. Choose the "Manual" setting and cook at High pressure for 8 minutes. Once cooking is complete, use a quick pressure release; carefully remove the lid.
4. Stir in corn kernels; seal the lid and allow it to sit in the residual heat until the corn is warmed through. Serve in individual bowls and enjoy!

Pork with Raisin and Port Sauce

Preparation Time: 35 minutes

Servings 6

Nutritional Values per serving: 395 Calories; 15.9g Fat; 21.4g Carbs; 40.9g Protein; 16.7g Sugars

Ingredients

- 1 tablespoon canola oil
- 2 pounds pork loin roast, boneless
- Kosher salt, to taste
- 1/2 teaspoon ground black pepper
- 1 teaspoon paprika
- 1/2 teaspoon mustard powder
- 1 teaspoon dried marjoram
- 2 cloves garlic, crushed
- 4 ounces raisins
- 1/2 cup port wine
- 1 cup pomegranate juice
- 1/2 teaspoon fresh ginger, grated

Directions

1. Press the "Sauté" button to preheat your Instant Pot. Now, heat the oil; sear the pork loin for 3 minutes on each side.

2. Then, add the remaining ingredients to your Instant Pot.
3. Secure the lid. Choose the "Poultry" setting and cook at High pressure for 15 minutes. Once cooking is complete, use a natural pressure release; carefully remove the lid.
4. Serve the pork topped with raisin-port sauce. Bon appétit!

Chipotle Pork with Salsa

Preparation Time: 35 minutes

Servings 6

Nutritional Values per serving: 398 Calories; 19.4g Fat; 8.1g Carbs; 45.5g Protein; 5.9g Sugars

Ingredients

- 1 ½ pounds pork loin, boneless and well-trimmed
- Kosher salt and ground black pepper, to your liking
- 1 teaspoon grainy mustard
- 1 (1-inch piece fresh ginger root, grated
- 1/3 teaspoon ground allspice
- 1/2 teaspoon ground bay leaf
- 2 tablespoons brown sugar
- 1 tablespoon chipotle paste
- 1 cup broth
- For the Salsa Sauce:
- 2 ripe tomatoes, peeled, seeds removed, chopped
- 2 tablespoons onion, finely chopped
- 1 clove garlic, minced
- 1mild chile pepper
- 2 tablespoons cilantro,chopped
- 1 ½ tablespoons lime juice
- Salt, to your liking

Directions

1. Sprinkle pork loin with all seasonings. Spritz the Instant Pot with a nonstick cooking spray.
2. Press the "Sauté" button to heat up your Instant Pot. Sear pork loin on both sides until just browned.
3. Add brown sugar, chipotle paste, andbroth. Secure the lid. Choose the "Manual" setting and cook for 25 minutes at High Pressure.
4. Once cooking is complete, use a natural release; remove the lid carefully.
5. Meanwhile, make the salsa by mixing all ingredients. Serve pork loin with fresh salsa on the side. Bon appétit!

Pork Carnitas Taquitos

Preparation Time: 1 hour

Servings 8

Nutritional Values per serving: 417 Calories; 24.4g Fat; 16.6g Carbs; 32.3g Protein; 11.8g Sugars

Ingredients

- 1 tablespoon lard, melted
- 2 pounds pork shoulder
- 1 tablespoon granulated sugar
- 1 teaspoon shallot powder
- 1 teaspoon granulated garlic
- Salt and black pepper, to taste
- 1 teaspoon ground cumin
- 1 cup ketchup
- 1 cup tomato paste
- 1/2 cup dry red wine
- 1 teaspoon mixed peppercorns
- 2 bay leaves
- 1 teaspoon chipotle powder
- 1/2 cup Manchego cheese, shredded
- 16 corn tortillas, warmed

Directions

1. Press the “Sauté” button to preheat your Instant Pot. Then, melt the lard. Sear the pork shoulder until it is delicately browned on all sides.
2. Add the sugar, shallot powder, garlic, salt, black pepper, cumin, ketchup, tomato paste, wine, peppercorns, bay leaves, and chipotle powder.
3. Secure the lid. Choose the “Meat/Stew” setting and cook at High pressure for 45 minutes. Once cooking is complete, use a natural pressure release; carefully remove the lid.
4. Shred the meat with two forks. Divide the shredded pork among tortillas. Top with cheese. Roll each tortilla and brush it lightly with oil.
5. Arrange tortillas on a cookie sheet. Bake approximately 13 minutes and serve. Enjoy!

Pork Chops with Creamed Mustard Sauce

Preparation Time: 15 minutes

Servings 4

Nutritional Values per serving: 433 Calories; 22.7g Fat; 7g Carbs; 48.3g Protein; 0.8g Sugars

Ingredients

- 2 tablespoons canola oil
- 4 pork loin chops
- Salt and ground black pepper, to taste
- 1 teaspoon smoked paprika
- 1/2 cup cream of celery soup
- 1/2 cup chicken broth
- 1 cup sour cream
- 1 tablespoon Dijon mustard

Directions

1. Press the "Sauté" button to preheat your Instant Pot. Then, heat the oil and sear the pork chops for 2 minutes per side.
2. Then, stir in salt, black pepper, paprika, cream of celery soup, andchicken broth.
3. Secure the lid. Choose the "Manual" setting and cook at High pressure for 9 minutes. Once cooking is complete, use a quick pressure release; carefully remove the lid.

4. Remove pork chops from the Instant Pot.
5. Fold in sour cream and Dijon mustard. Press the "Sauté" button again and let it simmer until the sauce is reduced and heated through. Bon appétit!

French-Style Pork and Bean Casserole

Preparation Time: 40 minutes

Servings 6

Nutritional Values per serving: 491 Calories; 27g Fat; 25.5g Carbs; 36.1g Protein; 7.1g Sugars

Ingredients

- 1 tablespoon olive oil
- 1 pound pork shoulder, cut into cubes
- 1/2 pound pork sausage, sliced
- 1 cup water
- 1 tablespoon beef bouillon granules
- 1 pound dry cannellini beans
- 1 cloves garlic, finely minced
- 1 yellow onion, sliced
- 1 parsnip, sliced
- 1 carrots, sliced
- 1 teaspoon celery seeds
- 1/2 teaspoon mustard seeds
- 1/2 teaspoon cumin powder
- Sea salt and ground black pepper, to taste
- 1 ½ cups sour cream

Directions

1. Press the “Sauté” button to preheat your Instant Pot. Heat olive oil until sizzling.
2. Then, brown the meat and sausage for 3 to 4 minutes, stirring periodically.
3. Add water, beef bouillon granules, cannellini beans, garlic, onion, parsnip, carrot, and seasonings.
4. Secure the lid. Choose the “Bean/Chili” setting and cook at High pressure for 30 minutes. Once cooking is complete, use a natural pressure release; carefully remove the lid.
5. Serve topped with sour cream. Enjoy!

Tender Aji Panca Pork

Preparation Time: 55 minutes

Servings 6

Nutritional Values per serving: 511 Calories; 30.7g Fat; 17.5g Carbs; 39.2g Protein; 16.4g Sugars

Ingredients

- 1 tablespoon lard
- 2 pounds pork shoulder
- 3/4 cup broth, preferably homemade
- 1/3 cup honey
- 2 tablespoons champagne vinegar
- 1 teaspoon garlic, minced
- 2 tablespoons soy sauce
- 1 teaspoon aji panca powder
- Kosher salt and ground black pepper, to your liking
- 1 tablespoon flaxseed, ground

Directions

1. Press the "Sauté" button, and melt the lard. Once hot, sear pork shoulder on all sides until just browned.
2. Add the broth, honey, vinegar, garlic, soy sauce, aji panca powder, salt, and pepper. Secure the lid. Select the "Manual" mode, High pressure and 50 minutes.

3. Once cooking is complete, use a natural release; remove the lid carefully. Set the pork shoulder aside keeping it warm.
4. Now, press the "Sauté" button again and add ground flaxseed to the cooking liquid. Let it simmer until the sauce has thickened.
5. Taste, adjust the seasoning and pour the sauce over the reserved pork shoulder. Bon appétit!

Southwestern-Style Cheese Meatloaf

Preparation Time: 35 minutes

Servings 6

Nutritional Values per serving: 352 Calories; 22.1g Fat; 13.2g Carbs; 24.8g Protein; 3.7g Sugars

Ingredients

- 1 pound ground pork
- 1 egg
- 1/2 cup scallions, minced
- 2 garlic cloves, minced
- 1/2 cup whole grain tortilla chips, finely crushed
- 1/2 cup Cotija cheese, crumbled
- Sea salt and ground black pepper, to taste
- 1 teaspoon smoked paprika
- 1 cup bottled chipotle salsa
- 2 tablespoons ketchup
- 1 teaspoon fresh lime juice

Directions

1. Prepare your Instant Pot by adding 1 cup of water and a metal rack to its bottom.
2. Thoroughly combine ground pork, egg, scallions, garlic, crushed tortilla chips, Cotija cheese, salt, black pepper, paprika, and 1/2 cup of salsa in a mixing bowl.

3. Now, shape the mixture into a meatloaf. Transfer the meatloaf to a lightly greased baking pan. Lower the baking pan onto the rack.
4. In a bowl, mix the remaining 1/2 cup of salsa with ketchup and lime juice. Brush the salsa mixture over top of the meatloaf.
5. Secure the lid. Choose the "Bean/Chili" setting and cook at High pressure for 30 minutes. Once cooking is complete, use a quick pressure release; carefully remove the lid. Bon appétit!

Easy Louisiana Ribs

Preparation Time: 30 minutes

Servings 6

Nutritional Values per serving: 365 Calories; 25g Fat; 3.7g Carbs; 3.1g Protein; 2.6g Sugars

Ingredients

- 2 pounds baby back ribs
- 2 slices fresh ginger
- 1/2 cup dry wine
- 1 tablespoon brown sugar
- 2 cloves garlic, sliced
- 2 tablespoons soy sauce
- 1 cup beef bone broth
- 1 teaspoon Cajun seasoning
- Sat, to taste

Directions

1. Add all of the above ingredients to your Instant Pot.
2. Secure the lid. Choose the "Meat/Stew" setting and cook at High pressure for 20 minutes. Once cooking is complete, use a natural pressure release; carefully remove the lid.
3. Serve warm and enjoy!

Pork Steaks Marchand de Vin

Preparation Time: 15 minutes

Servings 6

Nutritional Values per serving: 330 Calories; 22.2g Fat; 1.7g Carbs; 28.7g Protein; 0.6g Sugars

Ingredients

- 1 tablespoon lard, melted
- 1 ½ pounds pork steaks
- 1 cup demi-glace
- 1/2 cup red wine
- 2 bay leaves
- Sea salt and ground black pepper, to taste
- 1 teaspoon dried oregano

Directions

1. Press the "Sauté" button to preheat your Instant Pot. Melt the lard. Now, sear the pork steaks approximately 3 minutes per side.
2. Add the remaining ingredients to the Instant Pot.
3. Secure the lid. Choose the "Manual" setting and cook at High pressure for 8 minutes. Once cooking is complete, use a quick pressure release; carefully remove the lid.
4. Press the "Sauté" button one more time and continue simmering until the cooking liquid has reduced by three-fourths. Bon appétit!

Filipino Pork Soup

Preparation Time: 40 minutes

Servings 4

Nutritional Values per serving: 444 Calories; 16.9g Fat; 42.2g Carbs; 31.6g Protein; 5.1g Sugars

Ingredients

- 2 tablespoons vegetable oil
- 3/4 pound bone-in pork chops
- 1/2 cup sweet onion, chopped
- 1 teaspoon fresh garlic, crushed
- 2 sweet peppers, deveined and chopped
- 4 potatoes, peeled and diced
- 2 carrots, trimmed and thinly sliced
- 1 parsnip, trimmed and thinly sliced
- 4 cups vegetable broth, preferably homemade
- Salt and freshly ground black pepper, to taste
- 1/2 teaspoon paprika
- 1 teaspoon dried thyme
- 1 (1/2-inch piece fresh ginger, grated
- 1 (1.41-ounce package tamarind soup base

Directions

1. Preheat your Instant Pot on “Sauté” setting. Then, heat the vegetable oil and brown pork chops for 4 minutes on each side.
2. Add the remaining ingredients and secure the lid. Choose the “Soup” mode and cook for 30 minutes at High pressure.
3. Once cooking is complete, use a natural pressure release; remove the lid carefully. Serve hot with toasted bread. Bon appétit!

Kid-Friendly Pork Sandwiches

Preparation Time: 50 minutes

Servings 6

Nutritional Values per serving: 480 Calories; 18.4g Fat; 30.1g Carbs; 45.1g Protein; 3.3g Sugars

Ingredients

- 2 teaspoons lard, at room temperature
- 2 pounds pork shoulder roast, rind removed, boneless
- 2 garlic cloves, chopped
- 1 (1-inch piece fresh ginger, peeled and grated
- 1 tablespoon maple syrup
- 1/4 cup dry red wine
- 1 cup water
- 1/2 tablespoon Worcestershire sauce
- Sea salt, to taste
- 1/3 teaspoon ground black pepper
- 2 sprig thyme
- 2 whole star anise
- 1 tablespoon arrowroot powder
- 12 soft lunch rolls, warmed
- 1 cup pickles, sliced

Directions

1. Press the "Sauté" button to preheat your Instant Pot. Now, melt the lard. Once hot, sear the pork shoulder roast for 3 minutes per side.
2. Add the garlic, ginger, maple syrup, wine, water, Worcestershire sauce, and seasonings to the Instant Pot.
3. Secure the lid. Choose the "Meat/Stew" setting and cook at High pressure for 45 minutes. Once cooking is complete, use a natural pressure release; carefully remove the lid.
4. Transfer the pork shoulder to a chopping board. Shred the meat and return it back to the Instant Pot.
5. Whisk the arrowroot powder with 2 tablespoons of water; press the "Sauté" button again and add the slurry. Let it simmer until thickened.
6. Assemble the sandwiches with pork and pickles. Bon appétit!

Pork Roast with Fresh Avocado Sauce

Preparation Time: 35 minutes

Servings 6

Nutritional Values per serving: 442 Calories; 26.4g Fat; 8.7g Carbs; 42.3g Protein; 1.4g Sugars

Ingredients

- 2 pounds pork roast, cut into cubes
- 1 cup water
- 1 tablespoon beef bouillon granules
- 1 tablespoon fish sauce
- 1 habanero pepper, minced
- 1/2 cup scallions, chopped
- 1 teaspoon ginger-garlic paste
- 2 teaspoons olive oil
- Freshly ground black pepper, to taste
- Avocado Sauce:
- 1 avocado, pitted and peeled
- 2 tablespoons mayonnaise
- 2 garlic cloves, pressed
- 1 tablespoon fresh lime juice

Directions

1. Add pork roast, water, beef bouillon granules, fish sauce, habanero pepper, scallions, ginger-garlic paste, olive oil, and ground black pepper to the Instant Pot.
2. Secure the lid. Choose the "Meat/Stew" setting and cook at High pressure for 30 minutes. Once cooking is complete, use a natural pressure release; carefully remove the lid.
3. Meanwhile, whisk all of the sauce ingredients in a mixing bowl. Serve with pork roast and enjoy!

Thai Pork Medallion Curry

Preparation Time: 15 minutes

Servings 4

Nutritional Values per serving: 286 Calories; 15.3g Fat; 5.8g Carbs; 30.5g Protein; 1.7g Sugars

Ingredients

- 2 teaspoons coconut oil
- 1 pound pork medallions
- 1/2 teaspoon cumin seeds
- 1 jalapeño pepper, seeded and minced
- 1 bay leaf
- 1 ½ tablespoons fish sauce
- 1 cup beef bone broth
- 2 cloves garlic, minced
- 2 tablespoons Thai green curry paste
- 1 tablespoon apple cider vinegar
- Salt and ground black pepper, to taste
- 1/2 teaspoon cayenne pepper
- Zest and juice of 1 lime

Directions

1. Press the "Sauté" button to preheat the Instant Pot. Heat the coconut oil. Once hot, sear the pork medallions for 2 to 3 minutes.

2. Add the remaining ingredients, including roasted seasonings.
3. Secure the lid. Choose the "Manual" setting and cook at High pressure for 8 minutes. Once cooking is complete, use a quick pressure release; carefully remove the lid.
4. Serve with basmati rice and enjoy!

Easy Pork Sliders

Preparation Time: 1 hour 10 minutes + marinating time

Servings 6

Nutritional Values per serving: 433 Calories; 18.8g Fat; 20.9g Carbs; 43.9g Protein; 6g Sugars

Ingredients

- 2 pounds pork loin roast, cut into cubes
- 4 cloves garlic, smashed
- 2 tablespoons fresh scallions, chopped
- 1/2 cup pineapple juice
- Salt and black pepper, to taste
- 1 teaspoon cayenne pepper
- 1/4 teaspoon mustard seeds
- 1/4 teaspoon cumin
- 1 ½ tablespoons olive oil
- 1 head fresh Iceberg lettuce, leaves separated
- 2 tablespoons Dijon mustard
- 6 dinner rolls

Directions

1. Place the pork, garlic, scallions, pineapple, juice, salt, black pepper, cayenne pepper, mustard seeds, and cumin in a mixing bowl; wrap with a foil and transfer to your refrigerator for 2 hours.

2. Press the "Sauté" button and heat olive oil. Now, cook the pork, working in batches, until it is well browned.
3. Secure the lid. Now, select the "Manual" mode, High pressure and 60 minutes. Once cooking is complete, use a natural release; carefully remove the lid.
4. Serve over dinner rolls, garnished with fresh lettuce and Dijon mustard. Bon appétit!

Five-Star Picnic Shoulder

Preparation Time: 50 minutes

Servings 4

Nutritional Values per serving: 288 Calories; 12.7g Fat; 6.1g Carbs; 35.2g Protein; 3.2g Sugars

Ingredients

- 1 ½ pounds pork picnic shoulder
- 1 teaspoon garlic powder
- 1/2 teaspoon cumin powder
- 1/4 teaspoon cinnamon, ground
- 1 teaspoon celery seeds
- 1 teaspoon oregano, dried
- Sea salt and ground black pepper, to taste
- 1/2 cup fresh orange juice
- 1 cup beef bone broth

Directions

1. Place all of the above ingredients in the Instant Pot.
2. Secure the lid. Choose the "Meat/Stew" setting and cook at High pressure for 45 minutes. Once cooking is complete, use a natural pressure release; carefully remove the lid.
3. Test for doneness and thinly slice the pork; transfer to a serving platter. Serve warm and enjoy!

223. Asian Shrimp Appetizer

Preparation time: 10 minutes

Cooking time: 4 minutes

Servings: 4

Ingredients:

- 1 pounds shrimp, peeled and deveined
- 2 tablespoons coconut aminos
- 3 tablespoons vinegar
- ¾ cup pineapple juice
- 1 cup chicken stock
- 3 tablespoons stevia

Directions:

1. Put shrimp, pineapple juice, stock, aminos and stevia in your instant pot, stir a bit, cover and cook on High for 4 minutes.
2. Arrange shrimp on a platter, drizzle cooking juices all over and serve as an appetizer.
3. Enjoy!

Nutritional Values per serving: Calories 172, fat 4, fiber 1, carbs 3, protein 20

Mediterranean Octopus Appetizer

Preparation time: 10 minutes

Cooking time: 16 minutes

Servings: 6

Ingredients:

- 1 octopus, cleaned and prepared
- 2 rosemary sprigs
- 2 teaspoons oregano, dried
- ½ yellow onion, chopped
- 4 thyme sprigs
- ½ lemon
- 1 teaspoon black peppercorns
- 3 tablespoons olive oil
- For the marinade:
- ¼ cup extra virgin olive oil
- Juice of ½ lemon
- 4 garlic cloves, minced
- 2 thyme sprigs
- 1 rosemary sprigs
- Salt and black pepper to the taste

Directions:

1. Put the octopus in your instant pot, add oregano, 2 rosemary sprigs, 4 thyme sprigs, onion, lemon, 3

tablespoons olive oil, peppercorns and salt, stir, cover, cook on High for 10 minutes, transfer to a cutting board, cool it down, separate tentacles and transfer them to a bowl.

2. Add ¼ cup olive oil, lemon juice, garlic, 1 rosemary sprigs, 2 thyme sprigs, salt and pepper, toss to coat and leave aside for 1 hour.
3. Place octopus on preheated grill over medium high heat, cook for 3 minutes on each side, arrange on a platter and serve.
4. Enjoy!

Nutritional Values per serving: Calories 162, fat 3, fiber 1, carbs 2, protein 7

Chinese Squid Appetizer

Preparation time: 10 minutes

Cooking time: 15 minutes

Servings: 4

Ingredients:

- 4 squid, tentacles from 1 squid separated and chopped
- 1 cup cauliflower rice
- 14 ounces fish stock
- 4 tablespoons coconut aminos
- 1 tablespoon mirin
- 2 tablespoons stevia

Directions:

1. In a bowl, mix chopped tentacles with cauliflower rice, stir well and stuff each squid with the mix.
2. Place squid in your instant pot, add stock, aminos, mirin and stevia, stir, cover and cook on High for 15 minutes.
3. Arrange stuffed squid on a platter and serve as an appetizer.
4. Enjoy!

Nutritional Values per serving: Calories 162, fat 2, fiber 2, carbs 3, protein 10

Simple Artichokes

Preparation time: 10 minutes

Cooking time: 15 minutes

Servings: 4

Ingredients:

- 4 big artichokes, trimmed
- Salt and black pepper to the taste
- 2 tablespoons lemon juice
- ¼ cup olive oil
- 2 teaspoons balsamic vinegar
- 1 teaspoon oregano, dried
- 2 garlic cloves, minced
- 2 cups water

Directions:

1. Add the water to your instant pot, add the steamer basket, add artichokes inside, cover and cook on High for 8 minutes.
2. In a bowl, mix lemon juice with vinegar, oil, salt, pepper, garlic and oregano and stir very well.
3. Cut artichokes in halves, add them to lemon and vinegar mix, toss well, place them on preheated grill over medium high heat, cook for 3 minutes on each

side, arrange them on a platter and serve as an appetizer.

4. Enjoy!

Nutritional Values per serving: Calories 162, fat 4, fiber 2, carbs 3, protein 5

Cajun Shrimp

Preparation time: 4 minutes

Cooking time: 3 minutes

Servings: 4

Ingredients:

- 1 cup water
- 1 pound shrimp, peeled and deveined
- ½ tablespoon Cajun seasoning
- 1 teaspoon extra virgin olive oil
- 1 bunch asparagus, trimmed

Directions:

1. Put the water in your instant pot, add steamer basket, add shrimp and asparagus inside, drizzle Cajun seasoning and oil over them, toss a bit, cover pot and cook on High for 3 minutes.
2. Arrange on appetizer plates and serve as an appetizer.
3. Enjoy!

Nutritional Values per serving: Calories 152, fat 2, fiber 3, carbs 8, protein 15

French Endives

Preparation time: 10 minutes

Cooking time: 7 minutes

Servings: 4

Ingredients:

- 4 endives, trimmed and halved
- Salt and black pepper to the taste
- 1 tablespoon lemon juice
- 1 tablespoon ghee

Directions:

1. Set your instant pot on Sauté mode, add ghee, heat it up, add endives, season with salt and pepper, drizzle lemon juice, cover pot and cook them on High for 7 minutes.
2. Arrange endives on a platter, drizzle some of the cooking juice over them and serve as an appetizer.
3. Enjoy!

Nutritional Values per serving: Calories 100, fat 3, fiber 2, carbs 7, protein 2

Endives and Ham Appetizer

Preparation time: 10 minutes

Cooking time: 20 minutes

Servings: 4

Ingredients:

- 4 endives, trimmed
- 1 cup water
- Salt and black pepper to the taste
- 1 tablespoon coconut flour
- 2 tablespoons ghee
- 4 slices ham
- ½ teaspoon nutmeg, ground
- 14 ounces coconut milk

Directions:

1. Add the water to your instant pot, add steamer basket, add endives inside, cover, cook them on High for 10 minutes, wrap them in ham and transfer them to a baking dish
2. Clean your instant pot, set it on simmer mode, add the ghee, heat it up, add coconut flour, milk, salt, pepper and nutmeg, stir and cook for 7 minutes.
3. Pour milk and nutmeg mix over endives, introduce them in preheated broiler and broil for 10 minutes.

4. Arrange on a platter and serve as an appetizer.
5. Enjoy!

Nutritional Values per serving: Calories 152, fat 3, fiber 3, carbs 6, protein 12

Eggplant Spread

Preparation time: 10 minutes

Cooking time: 10 minutes

Servings: 6

Ingredients:

- 2 pounds eggplant, peeled and cut into medium chunks
- Salt and black pepper to the taste
- ¼ cup olive oil
- 4 garlic cloves, minced
- ½ cup water
- 3 olives, pitted and sliced
- ¼ cup lemon juice
- 1 bunch thyme, chopped
- 1 tablespoon sesame seed paste

Directions:

1. Set your instant pot on sauté mode, add oil, heat it up, add eggplant pieces, stir and cook for 5 minutes.
2. Add garlic, water, salt and pepper, stir, cover, cook on High for 3 minutes, transfer to a blender, add sesame seed paste, lemon juice and thyme, stir and pulse really well.
3. Transfer to bowls, sprinkle olive slices on top and serve as an appetizer.

4. Enjoy!

Nutritional Values per serving: Calories 87, fat 4, fiber 2, carbs 6, protein 2

Okra Bowls

Preparation time: 10 minutes

Cooking time: 15 minutes

Servings: 6

Ingredients:

- 1 pound okra, trimmed
- 6 scallions, chopped
- 3 green bell peppers, chopped
- Salt and black pepper to the taste
- 2 tablespoons olive oil
- 1 teaspoon stevia
- 28 ounces canned tomatoes, chopped

Directions:

1. Set your instant pot on Sauté mode, add oil, heat it up, add scallions and bell peppers, stir and cook for 5 minutes.
2. Add okra, salt, pepper, stevia and tomatoes, stir, cover, cook on High for 10 minutes, divide into small bowls and serve as an appetizer salad.
3. Enjoy!

Nutritional Values per serving: Calories 121, fat 3, fiber 3, carbs 6, protein 4

Easy Leeks Platter

Preparation time: 10 minutes

Cooking time: 10 minutes

Servings: 4

Ingredients:

- 4 leeks, washed, roots and ends cut off
- Salt and black pepper to the taste
- 1/3 cup water
- 1 tablespoon ghee

Directions:

1. Put leeks in your instant pot, add water, ghee, salt and pepper, stir, cover and cook on High for 5 minutes.
2. Set the pot on sauté mode, cook leeks for a couple more minutes, arrange them on a platter and serve as an appetizer.
3. Enjoy!

Nutritional Values per serving: Calories 73, fat 3, fiber 4, carbs 9, protein 7

Tomatoes Appetizer

Preparation time: 10 minutes

Cooking time: 10 minutes

Servings: 4

Ingredients:

- 4 tomatoes, tops cut off and pulp scooped
- ½ cup water
- Salt and black pepper to the taste
- 1 yellow onion, chopped
- 1 tablespoon ghee
- 2 tablespoons celery, chopped
- ½ cup mushrooms, chopped
- 1 cup cottage cheese
- ¼ teaspoon caraway seeds
- 1 tablespoon parsley, chopped

Directions:

1. Set your instant pot on sauté mode, add ghee, heat it up, add onion and celery, stir and cook for 3 minutes.
2. Add tomato pulp, mushrooms, salt, pepper, cheese, parsley and caraway seeds, stir, cook for 3 minutes more and stuff tomatoes with this mix.

3. Add the water to your instant pot, add the steamer basket, and stuffed tomatoes inside, cover and cook on High for 4 minutes.
4. Arrange tomatoes on a platter and serve as an appetizer.
5. Enjoy!

Nutritional Values per serving: Calories 152, fat 2, fiber 4, carbs 6, protein 7

Cinnamon and Pumpkin Muffins

Preparation time: 10 minutes

Cooking time: 20 minutes

Servings: 18

Ingredients:

- 4 tablespoons ghee
- ¾ cup pumpkin puree
- 2 tablespoons flaxseed meal
- ¼ cup coconut flour
- ½ cup erythritol
- ½ teaspoon nutmeg, ground
- 1 teaspoon cinnamon powder
- ½ teaspoon baking powder
- ½ teaspoon baking soda
- 1 and ½ cups water
- 1 egg

Directions:

1. In a bowl, mix ghee with pumpkin puree, egg, flaxseed meal, coconut flour, erythritol, baking soda, baking powder, nutmeg and cinnamon, stir well and divide into a greased muffin pan.

2. Add the water to your instant pot, add the steamer basket, add muffin pan inside, cover pot and cook on High for 20 minutes.
3. Arrange muffins on a platter and serve as a snack.

Nutritional Values per serving: Calories 50, fat 3, fiber 1, carbs 2, protein 2

Spicy Chili Balls

Preparation time: 10 minutes

Cooking time: 5 minutes

Servings: 3

Ingredients:

- 3 bacon slices
- 1 cup water
- 3 ounces cream cheese
- ¼ teaspoon onion powder
- Salt and black pepper to the taste
- 2 jalapeno peppers, chopped
- ½ teaspoon parsley, dried
- ¼ teaspoon garlic powder

Directions:

1. Set your instant pot on sauté mode, add bacon, cook for a couple of minutes, transfer to paper towels drain grease and crumble it.
2. In a bowl, mix cream cheese with jalapenos, bacon, onion, garlic powder, parsley, salt and pepper, stir well and shape balls out of this mix.
3. Clean the pot, add the water, and the steamer basket, add spicy balls inside, cover and cook on High for 2 minutes.

4. Arrange balls on a platter and serve as an appetizer.
5. Enjoy!

Nutritional Values per serving: Calories 150, fat 5, fiber 1, carbs 2, protein 5

Italian Dip

Preparation time: 10 minutes

Cooking time: 20 minutes

Servings: 4

Ingredients:

- 4 ounces cream cheese, soft
- ½ cup mozzarella cheese
- ¼ cup coconut cream
- Salt and black pepper to the taste
- 1/2 cup tomato sauce
- 4 black olives, pitted and chopped
- ¼ cup mayonnaise
- ¼ cup parmesan cheese, grated
- 1 tablespoon green bell pepper, chopped
- 6 pepperoni slices, chopped
- ½ teaspoon Italian seasoning
- 2 cups water

Directions:

1. In a bowl, mix cream cheese with mozzarella, coconut cream, mayo, salt and pepper, stir and divide this into 4 ramekins.
2. Layer tomato sauce, parmesan cheese, bell pepper, pepperoni, Italian seasoning and black olives on top,

3. Add the water to your instant pot, add the steamer basket, add ramekins inside, cover and cook on High for 20 minutes.
4. Serve this dip warm with veggie sticks on the side.
5. Enjoy!

Nutritional Values per serving: Calories 250, fat 15, fiber 4, carbs 4, protein 12

Avocado Dip

Preparation time: 10 minutes

Cooking time: 2 minutes

Servings: 4

Ingredients:

- ¼ cup erythritol powder
- 1 cup water
- ½ cup cilantro, chopped
- 2 avocados, pitted, peeled and halved
- ¼ teaspoon stevia
- Juice from 2 limes
- Zest of 2 limes, grated
- 1 cup coconut milk

Directi ons:

1. Add the water to your instant pot, add the steamer basket, add avocado halves, cover and cook on High for 2 minutes.
2. Transfer to your blender, add lime juice and cilantro and pulse well.
3. Add coconut milk, lime zest, stevia and erythritol powder, pulse again, divide into bowls and serve.
4. Enjoy!

Nutritional Values per serving: Calories 150, fat 6, fiber 2, carbs 4, protein 2

Minty Shrimp Appetizer

Preparation time: 10 minutes

Cooking time: 20 minutes

Servings: 16

Ingredients:

- 2 tablespoons olive oil
- 10 ounces shrimp, cooked, peeled and deveined
- 1 tablespoons mint, chopped
- 2 tablespoons erythritol
- 1/3 cup blackberries, ground
- 11 prosciutto slices
- 1/3 cup veggie stock.

Directions:

1. Wrap each shrimp in prosciutto slices and drizzle oil over them.
2. In your instant pot, mix blackberries with mint, stock and erythritol, stir, set on simmer mode and cook for 2 minutes.
3. Add steamer basket, and wrapped shrimp, cover pot and cook on High for 2 minutes.
4. Arrange wrapped shrimp on a platter, drizzle mint sauce all over and serve.
5. Enjoy!

Nutritional Values per serving: Calories 175, fat 6, fiber 2, carbs 1, protein 8

Zucchini Appetizer Salad

Preparation time: 10 minutes

Cooking time: 6 minutes

Servings: 4

Ingredients:

- 1 cup mozzarella, shredded
- ¼ cup tomato sauce
- 1 zucchini, roughly sliced
- Salt and black pepper to the taste
- A pinch of cumin, ground
- A drizzle of olive oil

Directions:

1. In your instant pot, mix zucchini with oil, tomato sauce, salt, pepper and cumin, toss a bit, cover and cook on High for 6 minutes.
2. Divide between appetizer plates and serve right away.
3. Enjoy!

Nutritional Values per serving: Calories 130, fat 4, fiber 2, carbs 4, protein 3

CPSIA information can be obtained
at www.ICGtesting.com
Printed in the USA
BVHW060226200722
642495BV00009B/611

9 781804 508602